Legacy for Donna

A Palliative Death Full of Blessings
A Plea for Preventive Health Genealogies

Denise Rodda, R.P.N.

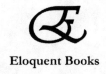

Eloquent Books

Eloquent Books
An imprint of Strategic Book Group
P.O. Box 333
Durham CT 06422
www.StrategicBookGroup.com

ISBN: 978-1-60911-589-0

Printed in the United States of America

I dedicate this book: of course, to my big sis Donna, Donna Ruth McCauley, Born: July 15, 1955 "DASH" September 17, 2008. To thank her for allowing me to care for her: to thank her for allowing me the privilege of being involved in the love and Blessings of her peaceful death. If allowed, I hope I am privileged enough to have loved ones 'fighting over who will spend time in bed with me,' hugging me as I die. And I also dedicate this story to another Donna; Donna Banks who passed of a mysterious, rapid cancer at the age of twenty-six. Today, her surviving family does not know what type of cancer this was. The tragedies and emotions of death sometimes make the details private, records are destroyed. To Donna Banks' sister, Nancey Stewart, who without her collaboration, this book would never have come to fruition. Thank you, My Friend; you are part of my 'Dash.' I also dedicate this to all those who do indeed remember to recognize their Blessings! To all those who will be enduring a death in palliative care—'Have it your way!' To all those who will be helping and loving them in this natural part of life!

Contents

Acknowledgments

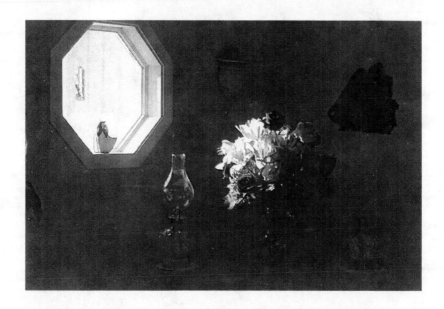

I Acknowledge:

Friends, patients and relatives for their support, whether it is knowing or unknowing, a part of the *Blessings* I experience daily.

I acknowledge the mysterious rainbows I see.

I must also acknowledge others lost, and thank them for their impact on my life: Linda Bull, Julie Fortin, Debbie Bruni, the child and Donna Banks.

Do they have a "what if?" story too?

Introduction

In retrospect, nursing my Big Sis Donna provided me with the hugest loving and spiritual experience I have ever been honoured with. Throughout her last eight days of life, my goal was to assist her to enjoy a peaceful death—she did. Some awe-inspiring occurrences took place; some big, some small. These occurrences led me to appreciate *Blessings* involved in death, and life.

My nursing career, experiences, and lessons learnt from other tragic deaths, other palliative deaths, taught me some vital life lessons. These prepared me to embrace this self-obligation I committed to. For others experiencing a palliative death, and their caregivers, their families, I wish to share and teach naturalness to this emotional and physical experience.

Donna was in the last stage of her cancer battle. I came to help. She entrusted me to be her confidant in death. Our family genealogy was discovered by medical science to be genetically positive for BRAC2. A discovered defect, called mutation, in our chromosomes predisposing us to the onset of cancer at an early age. I have been told I have a 99.9% chance of getting breast cancer and 30% likelihood of having ovarian cancer. Ovarian cancer is the deadlier cancer of the two.

Both of my sisters have had breast cancer. Darlene, the middle sister, is an eighteen year breast cancer survivor. It was finally discovered that our genealogy had an overwhelming number of women diagnosed with breast cancer. All having been diagnosed with this in their 30's and 40's: a very strong health genealogy. Donna never knew this history. Our immediate family health history, the history of our parents, has no breast or ovarian cancer diagnosis in it. Our father's sister is a breast cancer survivor. Paternal grandmother's three sisters had been the cancer victims. It had been hard to discover the truth about grandmother's sister's causes of death. Back then, early 1930ish, this female subject was not openly discussed.

Donna had both breast and ovarian cancer, and more. It spread to her kidney, abdomen, colon, bladder, skin, and lungs.

I am now enjoying late middle age, cancer-free. I have never had cancer. I have been offered and have undertaken a host of medical preventive treatments, as has my sister Darlene. Donna learned of this genetic predisposition only after her cancer had progressed to the more deadly ovarian cancer. It now would not have made any changes in her treatment options at this stage of the disease. The plea of *Legacy for Donna* is for society to make health genealogies. And to ensure young adults, in their formative years, learn to make their lifestyle choices with this knowledge. Not when disease strikes us!

Legacy for Donna will be your family health genealogy and your family living healthier; living longer. The lesson Donna's blessed, peaceful death can teach us all. I pray your family does not have "what ifs?" in its future.

Part I: Getting There

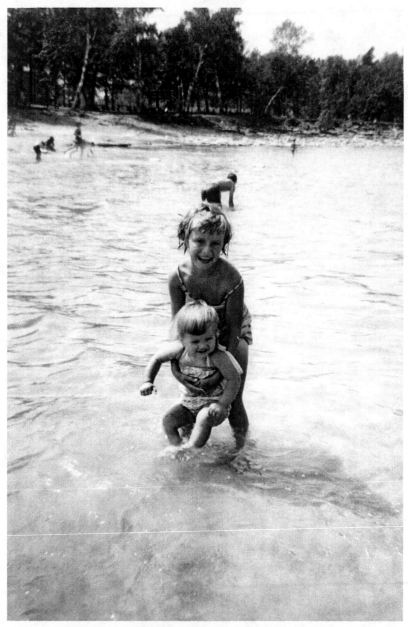

Donna and Denise—ages six and one.

1

Leading up to September 8th, Monday

I packed my bags last week. Anxious and munching like crazy for the past month, since my last visit to meet Wyman. Donna couldn't talk for the first two days of my visit, waiting for the long weekend to be over. She was afraid of being admitted to the emergency room again—palliative care. Her daughter, Erin, gave her mother a miracle visit with her newborn baby, Wyman, that first week in August.

I had received a birthday card from my Mom which included a $100 cheque and a message saying, "come visit." My wonderful boss, a general practitioner, M.D., was taking the week off so I was able to set aside my nurse responsibilities as well. My sister was getting significantly sicker—

trying to accept palliative care. Trying to accept death— hers—trying to accept that the doctors would give her no further treatment. She was now confiding in me by telephone and email.

Donna had been battling cancer for twelve years. She lived for all the treatments while holding onto hope. She eventually found her way back to Mom during the last five years of this illness, for nurturing. Her husband was strong and stoic in his own private world of tragedy. Losing his life mate; only being allowed to assist as much as she would permit. Emotional times! My sister's anger made her stronger to fight. She could be bitchy; we're sisters, so of course I knew. Denial, anger, bargaining, depression, and acceptance are the five stages of death, according to Elisabeth Kübler-Ross. Nurses are taught these stages. A terminal patient may go through each of these stages many times over, especially throughout a twelve-year fight with cancer. Since then, I have learned the three emotional stages of death:

1. Withdrawal, bargaining, anger, i.e. not visiting with others unless properly attired. Angry at herself for not being able to perform her own house keeping. Bargaining for further treatment.

2. Disbelieving, wondering, and doing, in order to make it real, i.e. giving possessions away to the proper person. Saying heartfelt thoughts to loved ones. Reminiscing of the wonder moments of their lives.

3. Supporting those around them to accept and allow them to die, i.e. no struggles with guilt for not being able to 'live' longer, no fault blaming, seeking God's guidance and peace.

I work in a medical practice with a husband and wife M.D. team. We share an office enjoying the fringe benefits of expression of love and appreciation on a daily basis from our patients (mainly Canadian-Italian). We work swiftly to try to accommodate the demands of a large practice in today's stressed medical system, year 2008.

My boss' wife, who also is a Palliative Care Doctor at our Sault Area Hospital Cancer Centre, said, "You should go." My boss, whom I credit with much wisdom and dedication to his patients and civic bonds of the Hippocratic Oath, said, 'I'll support you on any of your decisions."

Everyone has a personal tragedy to live with. You gain perspective while being a Physician's Assistant. I've been to funerals for children as young as four years old, supporting and receiving support from a past employer, a Paediatrician.

I worked for 14 months with a very special friend and nurse, Linda Bull. We job shared while she was going through her battle with cancer. In fact, we had been co-workers on the surgical floor at Sault Area Hospitals. We nursed together 15 years before, a friend then too. She was candid about her disease and loving to others always. She wore a sparkly make-up base which she called 'Angel Dust.' I think she did this to give herself strength to disguise the pallor treatment brings. We united as a team with a dedicated exemplary M.D. Linda passed away a couple of years ago. Her funeral service had standing room only. We nurses wore our uniforms. Even with support from precious nursing friends, I quietly cried during this service. I had too! Linda was a wonderful person, a loving mother and her love was unconditional. Her son gave me a Mother's Day Card one year, as I have no children of my own. Linda supported the entire oncology department, making friendships with others going through treatment. She hosted a girls' hotel and spa weekend with the prerequisite that no one was to mention the 'Cancer' word. I somehow knew that working with Linda would prepare me in life for other battles, my sister's battle, and my family's battle—my gift from Linda Bull!

Other friends had touched my life with their battles with cancer. I had known Julie Fortin, a scheduling clerk at the Group Health Centre for twenty years. We attended the same vegetarian cooking class. We had been 'Debbie fatties' together. Debbie Bruni was the Occupational Health Nurse, former scheduling clerk, who held morning weigh-ins and provided health tips to inspire and motivate staff at the Group Health Centre.

Julie was in remission from a form of cancer, called malignant melanoma, at the time I tested genetically BRAC 2 positive for cancer. My sister, Donna, consented to be genetically tested confirming where the chromosome mutation was on her D.N.A. cells. This allowed science to easily map and find this area in my blood sample. A part of our chromosomes had a hereditary defective called a mutation, for breast cancer, genetically predisposed, every cell in our body affected. This news threw my life into turmoil, but also saved my life. I got through this with support of some precious friends; Carol, Laurie, and Carole—the circle of friends. I cannot thank them enough for the emotional support they gave while I learned of the medical preventive and prophylactic treatments I could endure; the studies available and being done currently. Ontario Health opened up an overwhelming host of options and choices. I had to learn where my comfort zone was. What I needed to do to save my life. I felt changed, was changed, and had to face some scary options. I'll dwell on what I learned later, and what I will continue to learn—to advise others, spread the word. Prevention is possible!

I heard about Julie's death from another co-worker in the morning. I was devastated, but did not get a chance to cry until around 9:30 p.m., as I had to keep going until the days tasks were done—sad and pathetic that demands on my life would not allow me time to feel.

Julie and I bonded with this cancer diagnosis. She shared glimpses of her personal treatments and shared her joy of being able to go to work, to not be sick, to forget about the bitching. I visited her in the hospital about one month before her death, at age fifty-two. Because her throat, mouth, and jaw were affected, I brought popsicles and magazines to her. I spoke briefly with her husband at the funeral. He remembered me as the "Popsicle Nurse." She left behind two young adult sons and a devoted husband. While going through the funeral line, something made me say to her sister-in-laws, "Please help and support these children." Perhaps I could envision being in their place. I knew I could.

Debbie Bruni's death took me by surprise. They had diagnosed her with lung cancer when confirming pneumonia just two Christmas holidays before. I thought gossip said they had caught it early. People said she was dropping into the office occasionally. I know the lung cancer chemo was a good treatment.

My sister had remised spectacularly with her lung cancer treatments. Her thoracentesis treatment progressed from weekly to three to four month intervals. We thought we had lost her the previous November/December. But Donna was fighting harder as her daughter had just announced her first pregnancy, due in June. As Donna fought even harder now, at times she was quite demanding. Her focus was to make it through another day to see her pregnant daughter. She only dreamt she'd be alive to see her new grandchild. Beating all odds, she not only got to see her pregnant daughter, she was able to see the baby more than once. She held the baby on her lap on her deathbed. She was called a "Miracle Patient" by her oncologists.

One of Debbie's sisters, Lori, is also a registered nurse at the Group Health Centre and a friend through my past twenty year nursing career. I saw Lori in Canadian Tire parking lot this spring. She spoke about praying that her sister had a 'good day.' I didn't realize at the time what she meant. I now understand the truth, the impact of that statement. I had gotten so busy with my own life and didn't hear the news that Debbie was being discharged from palliative care until it was too late. I was thinking, 'I'll visit soon, or do something.' I learned about Debbie's death from my scheduling clerk Jean. Such a wonderful, competent, exemplary women—a friend by employment and a friend of a friend too! Our northern town is like that!

I was madly cleaning Cedar View Cottage with its grand season opening scheduled for the next day, Saturday. My father-in-law Ron, his wife Nancy, and nieces and nephews Chandler, Chase, Carly, Jordan, Sierrah, and Alexandra, were up for their yearly Canadian trip. I had booked a week's holidays to pace my cottage work and to allow for family visiting. Now a family tradition, so the kids and Grandpa tell us!

Jean had phoned me at Cedar View Cottage to advise me of a change in a scheduled shift. She informed me of Debbie's passing. I was shocked. The visitation was that evening. The funeral home was on the ride home and I wanted to go. I had to go, for myself, my acceptance, for Debbie's sister, Lori, and for any other Group Health Centre staff and friends. I sent my family back to our home on River Road and told my husband what I had to do. I wouldn't be long. I had supper coordinated at home. I tried to clean up. I think I was cleaning the oven, fridge, and bathroom. I know I looked bad, wearing a sweatshirt and jeans. My hair was up in a clip from cleaning. I tried to freshen up my face and look presentable before I left. I arrived at the funeral home to be told that the visitation line was two hours long! I panicked as I couldn't wait two hours. I had the family at home to feed.

I spotted a friend and co-worker, Elaine, who was also a confidante about cancer. Her best friend had battled mastectomy while my sister was at the chemo stage. We had worked side by side. She is a most competent colleague, a caring cardiology nurse. I worked for another dedicated physician then. He was dedicated to his patients, his family and to his obligation to living and enjoying life. I thought of him as a friend. I liked his priorities and humour to get through life's stresses. I told Elaine of my predicament. Bless her heart, she advised me to go on up the line to see if I could see someone else from the Group Health Centre and join the line further up. Whether I wasn't seeing straight or not thinking, I loved the idea but couldn't find anyone else from our organization. I went before the Registry and asked if I could please butt in line. The gracious fellow mourners were only too happy to accommodate me. I signed the registry and joined the family receiving line. Debbie's family was graciously shaking hands and sharing hugs. How can they keep the strength to endure this?, I thought. I met Debbie's mother and told her my fifty-two year old sister was also battling cancer. I said, "God bless" and she said it back to me.

When I saw Lori, she graciously thanked me for coming. I stuttered an explanation about my attire, but said I had to come. Lori had the grace and composure to say, "Debbie always thought highly of you." How could she be strong enough to support me? A hug. I shared our similarities with my sister battling cancer too. I needed to share a moment of 'sisterhood' with her and told her to call me if I could help. I raced home to my duties, changed and *Blessed* from this experience. I do laugh; I never thought I would butt into line at a funeral. So bold, 'bold as brass' as my late Grandmother Ashworth would say. You do whatever you need to do to work things out. Faith, God rules always.

I had discussed these deaths with my sister. Not until there was no further treatment available and she was on the phone crying. I asked her if she had ever seen anyone die? I said that I had and it was OK. I shared the other young deaths with her. She hadn't known anyone else in this predicament, this cancer battle. In sharing, I had hoped to help her feel not so isolated. Fighting so hard can make a person feel alone. She seemed to gain comfort from this. I said, 'I never thought I would be having a conversation like this with you. Never!' She seemed to give me the responsibility of helping her mentally prepare to die after this. It happened then. Before this, our visits were for support; laughter to assist with stress relief; to share memories and to make memories. I always said I'd come visit her anytime she needed me. I was only a one and a half hour flight away. I could never accept a visit as potentially being my 'last visit' with my big sis Donna. For her sake and mine; I couldn't accept it.

The first week of August 2008, I flew down to visit Donna on Sunday after my Saturday cottage cleaning was done. Mom and Len picked me up at the airport. Then I met baby Wyman, with Erin my niece, and shared a family reunion that my sister thought she'd never live to see. A week visiting with her daughter, her grandbaby, Mom, Len, my sister Darlene and husband Wolfgang and their youngest daughter, Jennifer. I had to leave the following Friday to prepare for my Saturday cottage cleaning so I missed meeting Erin's new partner, Brian, and my niece, Amanda.

I made a family and baby video featuring a song by Carrie Underwood. "Sometimes that mountain you've been climbing is just a grain of sand. You find what you've been searching for is in your hand": the lesson in the background. Brother-in-law Jeff burned copies for everyone. It made everyone cry. Because Donna was sick, she couldn't join us on Mom's porch while baby Wyman was being shown off. When she did hold the baby, he enjoyed her comfort. There was a natural bond—Granny and Grandson. Donna said she wanted to be called Granny just like in the "Beverly Hillbillies" old TV program!

She had a thoracentesis on Tuesday, and later that week, was even able to get out of the house to Mom's for dinner. I drove her in her golf cart to watch a shuffleboard tournament that her husband and our mother were in. They needed outlets with friends. The pressure of Donna's illness was weighing heavily on both Mom and Donna's husband, Jeff. Each had their own health concerns also. I took Donna for a golf cart drive by the beach and then back home. I found out later she'd been too sick to go out. Or was she withdrawing from life? She hadn't been to the clubhouse or beaches at all this past month, July. My visit ended with a drive back to the airport with my brother-in-law Jeff, Donna's husband. We shared and talked and found the two-hour ride was too short.

On this "one last" visit with Donna she allowed me to enter her private world of dying, living and loving. To watch and be part of her beautiful gracious death! I think Donna means 'full of grace.' Mom says it means 'lady.' She was both! Denise means 'goddess of wine' and 'entertainer.' I was both. Thus, all of August that year, I was anxious and sick with worry. I watched and revised the video I had made, to do something for Donna. In fact this was therapeutic for me. I needed to do something for her! She was declining. She got a fever and was hospitalized for ten days. She began needing thoracentesis, lung draining and paracentesis, abdominal fluid draining again: Every four to five days. Donna also had palliative abdominal radiation treatment in the Whitby Hospital that month. Now it was early September, how could so much have gone on? How could I tell what was really happening? That's when I started to appreciate the miracles of *Blessings* which led me to make "one last" visit to help Donna, Mom, and Jeff.

I was anxious for another reason that September in 2008. Mom was scheduled for a colonoscopy, a scope test, to investigate abdominal concerns. Could it be cancer or a bleeding ulcer, a result of the constant worry of Donna's illness over the past five years? If they found anything notorious, they would tell Mom at this Wednesday's appointment. I was frantic. Donna was scheduled to have her, thoracentesis, lungs drained that Friday. Who would help her if Mom wasn't in the picture? Who would help Mom? I called Mom on Tuesday and told her my fears. She promised to call me with her test results as soon as possible. She didn't want me to come for a visit then. I called Donna and she said yes she was sick, but she'd rather I came to help her dress, attend and organize her son's engagement party on September twentieth. But would she be alive then? I waited, but had packed my suitcase so I would feel ready, just in case. My sister, Darlene, would be there within two hours, if needed. Although Darlene is talented and strong minded, her emotional talents could not be the equivalent of mine—a trained nurse with death experience. Or maybe it's my ego—only I could help. Or maybe it's my selfishness. I needed the security of being there instead of dealing with the anxiety over what's happening today? Is she having a good day? Just like Lori spoke of.

My father had battled debilitating heart disease since I was fifteen years old. He died on September 8th, 1993 when I was thirty-two years old. As I was the last child at home, I had forged a special bond with my mother through despair, illness, support, and then grief. Another tragedy and another story! I loved my father. He taught me many things and I can say that I am proud to be like him.

I'd missed my father's last three months of life. Jamie my husband and I were managing an isolated fly in fishing lodge eighteen hours north of their home then. It had been impossible to visit. I needed to "be there" for Donna. I needed to "be there" for me, this time.

I cleaned cottages that Saturday and had the *Blessing* of two cottages being reserved for 'month long rentals.' I now wasn't tied to home due to my cottage housekeeping tasks. My advertising and correspondence duties could be done from anywhere, thanks to the beauty of internet services. This was *Blessing # one*, as the cottage housekeeping would normally be done on a weekly basis. I was now freed from one job.

On my way to clean the cottages, I habitually tried to give myself extra time to drive through town and go to a couple of garage sales on route to the cottages. That Saturday I found a soft beanbag neck support and a black lace shawl for $1.00 each. I bought them hoping they would come in handy one day. I also bought bath bubbles scented in violet rose. Donna gained physical comfort in the bath. At times needing three to four soothing baths a day for relief.

I had been a bit 'more blonde' in August, due to my anxiety for Donna. I lost my driving glasses and was using a broken, scratched old pair. Another *Blessing!* While cleaning cottages, I found a pair of glasses and low and behold, they were a perfect prescription; better than mine! Although I looked like a librarian wearing them, my vanity could deal with this. Now I was road and travel ready.

On my way home from cottage cleaning that Saturday, I stopped at a friend's house to drop off some summer beach wear they had left at our house. These good people, Cooki and Al allowed me to vent my anxiety. I found it harder to do this with my husband, Jamie. I had made four 'emergency trips' to see Donna in the past two years when she had had significant health declines and battles. He did not realize nor have my nursing knowledge base, to understand that this time things were different. Palliative care, no further treatments could stop or remiss her cancer! Donna was wasting away, turning into a ghost of a person. I had thought in the past that perhaps Donna would have a health event, a complication, and pass away quickly. Perhaps she would not make it to the hospital emergency department in time. Congestive heart failure, kidney failure, lungs, and abdomen constantly filling up and not being able to breathe—a million different possible ways for sudden death to conquer her. She kept fighting, kept managing her symptoms. In doing so, she prolonged her quality of life and her length of life. She had seen that newborn grandson!

Her son, David, living in Kentucky, had just announced his engagement and planned a November 15th wedding. The doctors told Donna and Jeff to make this sooner if David's Mom was to participate. An engagement party was planned for September 20th, at the Victoria Place Clubhouse, for the new Kentucky family to meet our family. Donna and Jeff enjoyed many daily phone calls from their son to plan and share his joy in this event. Donna had met and loved David's fiancée, Kathy, from the start. They are a great couple.

Family members were concerned regarding the September twentieth party. Donna is now too sick to go. She cannot sit for more than half an hour. She is getting weaker by the day. How can they be planning an engagement party? Leave it to my sister to make her last "job in life," planning a family party! I respected her for this. Leave it be. God and fate will help us sort this out. It could be cancelled anytime if need be. Donna wants this. Let's continue to give her pleasure knowing we support this engagement party.

But I wanted to go help them now! Mom and Jeff both are exhausted from the last years of intense cancer treatments and support. Both devoted their existence to supporting Donna.

Now Donna did not want me to visit for Mom's September fourth scope test as she said she needed me later in the month to help her get ready (dress, plan) for the engagement party on September twentieth.

September twentieth might as well have been years away. So much had happened so quickly in her health's decline this last month of August. She was already too sick to attend a party from what Mom had told me.

I planned a visit, leaving this Friday, as my M.D. was off on a vacation then. I called Donna and told her I was coming. I was too anxious to stay home until September twentieth!

Jeff had taken an early retirement five years ago, due to multiple heart concerns and now was also battling diabetes. He told me in confidence that he was using his nitro spray for angina, more and more. He wouldn't tell Donna or Mom. I had to 'work' the information out of him as only a bratty little sister can!

My girlfriend, Cooki, phoned me the next day, Sunday. She advised to me to go before Wednesday if I wanted to see my sister alive! I asked, "You had a premonition?" Her response, "Yes, I just need to tell you this. Do what you want with this information. It is up to you." Now I was extremely anxious for Friday and my planned trip to come!

At work the next day, Monday, I arranged to be off the following week. I was even more anxious now. Donna was having a thoracentesis today, Monday. She had been so short of breath when I last spoke to her two days ago. She could barely talk.

As soon as I got home from work, Monday, I called Mom. How did it go? They had had an exhausting miserable experience taking Donna to the hospital in a rainstorm. Donna was able to get to the department only by wheelchair. She became drenched on the way through the parking lot. Thank goodness that the staff knew Donna and she was always treated spectacularly there. They took her immediately for her thoracentesis.

Now she was home, exhausted, sleeping, and still needing the oxygen!

I called Auntie Joan, my late father's sister, who is a forty-year breast cancer survivor. She and my Uncle John had seen Donna on Sunday for a short visit. Auntie Joan said she had been in tears since this visit. She told me Uncle John, too, had been crying.

Too anxious to sleep myself, I thought I'd make a quick call to Donna to wish her good night. As she was sleeping and exhausted, I spoke with Jeff at length. I then called my husband, Jamie, to listen on the phone as well. He had to hear this conversation in order to understand. Jeff explained that Donna was having disoriented times, incoherent at times, but clearly getting more chronic daily. Jeff relayed, "Every time the phone rings, or she hears the front door, she says, is that Denise on the phone? Is that Denise at the door?" This broke my heart.

I went to bed and thought. I decided to call in sick the next day, Tuesday; too stressed and anxious to focus on work. I would travel the next day (Tuesday) to Bobcageon and the Victoria Place subdivision where Donna and Mom lived. I could not wait until Friday!

Tuesday, September eighth was the anniversary of our Father's death, 17 years ago. I'm likely superstitious but I wondered if Donna would 'pass' on that day too. Being a nurse, I had heard of this happening only too often. I asked Jeff if Donna knew what Tuesday stood for. Yes, Mom had mentioned it—oh no!!

All things played on my mind at bedtime that night. Cooki's warning, Dad's death and the heartbreaking echo of Donna asking, "Is that Denise?" I will tell Jamie in the morning, no matter what, I had to go Tuesday!

2

September 9th, Tuesday

I called work and told my scheduling clerk I was in no shape for work! I finished my packing. I even vacuumed my car, which I called my truck. I leave the back seat down to make a 'dog house' for Kayla our Black Labrador Retriever, in the trunk and also keep miscellaneous cleaning supplies and tool boxes on hand. It was in a constant mess.

Jamie supported my decision to go but was worried sick about me driving by myself. I called my Nurse Practitioner's assistant, my friend Laurie. I had advised them earlier of the weight of stress I was feeling due to Donna's illness. "God bless and be careful. We'll give you a week off, then reassess—just phone us." How wonderful not to have an extra financial worry. I was stressed and couldn't focus on work. I needed to 'nurse' my sister, to be with her. I needed to try to support Mom and Jeff also. I could tell that the strain was taking its toll on them both: Anxiety, fatigue and worry.

When I was ready with car packed, almost out the door, I called Donna's house. Donna answered!! She started talking about a phone call regarding a medical appointment. She had spoken on the phone moments earlier and now couldn't remember who or what the purpose of this phone call was. Her mind, memory, thought process was jumbled. Likely from the morphine and I think from focusing so hard on just surviving. I told her I was coming to visit today, not waiting for Friday. She replied, "Oh Really!" "Yes, I'm almost out the door. Don't worry until 10:00 p.m. tonight. Don't tell Mom until later today as she will worry all day. I'll come straight to your house." I had hoped that her knowing I was on my way, she would 'hang on' today! I'd keep worrying until 12:00 midnight passed—until the dreaded 'Death Anniversary" of my father had passed. My girlfriend's premonition was still playing on my mind.

Finally, with the tires and fluids checked on the car, Kayla and I were on our way. Kayla, our old diabetic, visually impaired dog was settled in the doghouse trunk. Jamie thought I would be safer travelling the ten hour drive with a big dog beside me. I thought, should Jamie need to fly down urgently for a funeral, Kayla would already be with me. No one but the two of us can manage the two insulin needles per day. At least, there is no one we wanted to impose this chore upon nor did we want to upset Kayla. She travels well.

I have been called a Doggy Diabetic Nurse and have been fortunate enough to assist other dog owners to regulate their pets' illnesses. So far, our Kayla has survived diabetes with its complications of cataracts, with two insulin shots per day, for five years. When we say, "it's medicine dog time," Kayla comes to our spot in the household and waits for her insulin needle. Of course, she gets her doggy treat for this behaviour. Kayla is a laidback, older, very intelligent dog! Is it possible to have gained strength from a dog? I'm sure it is!

We had a good travelling day. I drove from one Tim Horton's Coffee Shop to another Tim Horton's Coffee Shop on the ten hour trip. We passed Blind River, Manitoulin Island, North Bay, Gravenhurst and several small towns and cottage country winding roads to Fenlon Falls. I

choose this scenic route, as it was in my comfort zone for driving, avoiding the Metropolis
of major highways with high-speed traffic. My
car should be in better shape. The electrical system was terribly messed up. Every trouble light
I had was on and had been for the past six
months. My gas gauge was also not working,
and something's up, my muffler sounds loud.
Driving carefully, not going over the speed
limit. I was grateful to have CAA back-up.
Please car; don't give out on me now!

It became a very dark evening. Close to
Donna's home, I took a wrong turn. The sign
said Old Highway 12. Is my map old? Yes, I'd
better take this turn. I kept my eyes peeled for
road signs. I was very aware of the dangers of
driving at night posed by deer and other animals
in that area. Watching and alert for glaring eyes
in the shadows of the roadside, I drove on. After
fifteen to twenty minutes, passing only cottages,
houses, forest and lakes, I saw a gas station. I
decided to stop and ask if my directions were
correct. "Nope, you got to go back and turn left
further up—no other way," the attendant
drawled. Now I was conscious that I may not
arrive before 10:00 p.m. and everyone would
start to worry. I did as the attendant had
directed. Eventually I was relieved to see the

sign Bobcageon—Yeah! The roads are looking familiar; the retirement subdivision called Victoria Place came into site, and then Donna and Jeff's driveway.

Mom came running out of the house, "I can't believe you're here!"

Part II: The Vigil

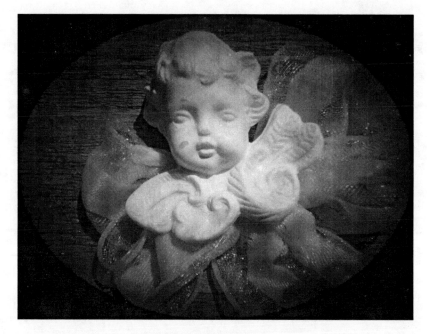

**My "Angel Promise," which mysteriously
fell off the fridge magnet.**

3

September 9th, Tuesday

Inside the house I found Jeff, and Len, Mom's companion, in the living room. Hugs! I then saw Donna sitting in her chair. Her favourite easy chaise, resting vertically made it easier to breathe, her homemade beautiful quilt from the Cancer Society on her lap. A different Donna from a month ago when I had last seen her! I had expected this, but now I could see. Sallow skin, bony wrists, withered away body and pale. The morphine pump was at her side. Her oxygen was constantly on. There was a humming made from this machine. We hugged and she said, "I'm alright, now you are here."

I had to give Kayla her medicine immediately.

Things get blurry for me now. I need to piece the next eight days together. I keep having 'flash backs' of moments, events, the days now run into each other. Stress and sleep deprivation start here.

I remember Donna saying, "I won't be able to talk to you much, I get so short of breath." I reply, "That's OK, you know I can do enough talking for the both of us!" I remember Donna being walked to the bathroom stating she was too tired and had to go to bed. Not strong enough to walk safely by herself. The oxygen and morphine pump line needing to be organized. I also remember Jeff preparing her pills. She took them happily and childlike, with her juice with ice through a straw—just how she always liked it. It had come to this had it!

I think I kissed her goodnight and she was tucked into bed by Mom and Jeff. Donna was set up in the computer room with a hospital bed, flowers, cards here and there, head up and pillows placed around her, to save her energy supporting herself.

I left with Mom and Len to go to their house, three doors away. I settled in their basement bedroom fondly nicknamed by my nieces, The Dungeon. It was the greatest room with two singles in it, dark with florescent glowing star stickers on the ceiling. A year or so before, I teased my mother saying I wanted to see the 'Big Dipper' in the night sky. She had now added more stars and indeed I slept under the ceiling's night's sky under the Big Dipper.

Daisy, my Mom's adopted Pug, was scaring Kayla. We laughed; Kayla had never seen anything 'snort' like that before. She looked at me as if to say "what is that?! I'm supposed to tolerate this? Let me hide from it!" As Kayla's vision was not the best, she could not confidently go down the steps. I carried my eighty-five pound dog down to The Dungeon.

Mom and I cried together that evening. Mom asked if the changes in Donna scared and shocked me. No, I was a nurse, I had anticipated this or maybe even worse. It was then that Mom told me why she was so shocked that I had arrived.

Mom and Len had dropped in on Donna around 8:30 that evening. In the past week of having the morphine pump, Donna's mind would occasionally wander. Illogical thoughts or memories would dominate until she 'focused' or until her body adjusted to the morphine. I had been told by Donna, that the morphine did take away the pain. In an earlier conversation, she said, "It was great, wish I'd had it sooner."

Donna always downplayed her symptoms, even with the doctors, as she didn't want to accept she was so sick and wanted to 'bargain' with the doctors for more treatment. Up until now, treatment had given her 'her life.' She was angry, frustrated and depressed when they told her there is no more treatment they could offer. Nothing they had in medical science was working now.

On my earlier visit in August, she had asked me what palliative care was. I told her it was to manage pain symptoms effectively, to prolong comfort and to prolong "Quality of Life." Managing your good times to allow you to do whatever is most important. We had discussed this on the phone, but she now needed to hear it again.

People seem to think that palliative care is a death sentence; a giving up, no hope. A very scary attitude! She needed to understand that palliative care meant more pain free quality time. Although symptoms would not go away, if controlled with modern medicine and the discipline to pace yourself, you could plan for the good moments of the day and rest pain free when needed. This would extend her life. Palliative care is giving maximum comfort and medical attention to each individual need.

In the first three or four days of my last visit with Donna, I did witness her mind wandering. Jeff and Mom knew she could not be left alone anymore, too weak and occasionally confused.

That evening, Mom recalled she had gotten a phone call last week at 1:00 a.m. Alarmed at such a late call, she jolted from bed to answer. It was Donna. She asked my Mom to send her husband back home so he could make supper! Mom gently explained that she would, and told Donna to lie down, rest and sleep. Mom was now having this new confusion symptom in the forefront of her mind.

Earlier tonight, when Mom and Len stopped in to "visit" Donna, Donna had said at 9:30 p.m., "that Denise should be arriving soon." Mom explained that Denise was coming Friday, three more days. At 9:45 p.m. Donna insisted that Mom call my husband, Jamie, in Sault Ste. Marie to see when I had left. Mom placated Donna by phoning, fully expecting me to answer the phone. Donna spoke with Jamie, rational but her speech slurred from the pain medication. Mom was shocked that Donna was correct! I then pulled into the driveway. Mom came running out, "I can't believe you're here." I did not understand her exuberance at that time. Wow, my sister kept a secret!!

As other family members arrived during the course of the next week, we could tease my sister Donna, about us not telling her of their travelling days. Some incredibly long drives were had. She would be worried sick and loose precious rest time or precious quality time with the stress of worry. Donna would not be upset with us over this as we explained it was 'pay back' time for her keeping Mom in the dark about my arrival. I had asked Donna on the phone that morning for her to wait only until later in the afternoon, before telling Mom of my expected arrival. Donna decided to "take it to the max" and tell Mom only one half hour before I was to arrive! Donna hadn't wanted my Mom to worry about my travelling alone, so indeed had kept this worry to herself and hubby all day. She was certainly aware of the important things, whether episodes of confusion did cloud her mind on occasion. Wow! This secret Donna kept also turned into another *Blessing*.

Mom told me that the home care nurse had advised Jeff to prepare funeral arrangements. Wow! The nurse advised Jeff of the confusion and added stress NOT having this done in advance would bring. Death was not immediate, but who knew? There were significant declines in Donna's strength and condition daily. Tomorrow at 1:00 p.m., Jeff and Mom planned to go to the funeral parlour to make these final arrangements. I would take care of Donna. Then Mom said that the last thing Donna said to her was 'don't you and Denise be up all night talking.' Her mind indeed 'worked' for things that were a priority!

It was past midnight when we finally did go to bed. I needed to ensure Donna did survive the full 24 hours of this anniversary day of my Father's death. I explained my premonitions to Mom. Perhaps this was a *Blessing* given to me by my late Father. This premonition and other occurrences (new glasses: Cooki's warning) which had helped me decide to travel three days earlier than planned. I am so happy I decided to come to her at this time.

Exhausted under the Big Dipper and overwhelmed, I allowed myself the peace of rest that night.

4

September 10th, Wednesday

I slept in; knowing the home care nurse from the Community Care Access Centre was coming in each morning. I would be in the way. I was anxious to spend some one-on-one with Donna. Did she know her funeral plans were being arranged today? No, I would go over to Donna's house and Donna would be told her husband Jeff had to go to run errands and do banking. What an incredibly stressful thing for Jeff and Mom to do.

Mom wanted to support Jeff. She also wanted to ensure that everything would be 'nice' for Donna. But mainly, I feel she needed to do this with my brother-in-law Jeff in order to help her accept Donna's fate. Donna would die soon. Mom was very teary, but was getting appropriately dressed and rallying her strength for this 'outing.' Although it broke my heart, I was very proud of her.

I showered and said I wanted to go to Donna's early to touch base with Jeff. How was he coping? I needed also to have an understanding of Donna's true condition before we were alone together. Kayla and I drove the three houses down the street. I brought garden tomatoes which were given to me by a generous, loving patient from Sault Ste. Marie. I also brought my garage sale bean bag neck pillow, so comfy and the violet bath bubbles.

I had assured Donna weeks earlier in a phone conversation that I would come nurse her when or if she needed me. She had been more concerned for me. How can you? You're so busy! I schemed a response for her, my husband and myself, indicating that I was not busy. I would love to enjoy the time while she was resting or sleeping by finally doing some of our business promotional projects on my laptop computer. I needed Donna to also feel free to do only what she felt up to and had energy for. To rest peacefully anytime she wanted to, while I sat with her. She didn't need to stress her body with visiting, entertaining me. I was pleased to just hang out and get some work done! She believed this. This would ease her obligations to me. As a 'big sis,' her will power would insist she fill this role, unless I assured her it would only be good for her to rest once in a while, whenever. It justified my trip for me and took some guilt away. It sounded very rational to me and a considering thought for my husband. I knew it was getting tough for Mom and Jeff.

I never realized that I would never be able to focus on anything else but Donna and the family for the next ten days. My strength and thought process would only allow for assessment, comprehension of Donna's health, ever changing planning—moment by moment, and the nursing of my sister.

Donna had actually forgotten that Mom had her colonoscopy, intestinal scope test scheduled last week. She and my Mom had both worried over this as the diagnosis could be colon cancer. Donna had only the strength to focus on making it through the day, catching her breath, waiting for the next scheduled thoracentesis while her lungs filled up with fluids, more and more each day; a terrible symptom resulting from her lung cancer. She was timing this procedure so she could have it done with the gentle expertise of the "Catheter Lab" at Peterborough's new hospital. They did it best. Once in Emergency, her lung had started bleeding and she had terrible pain after Emergency Room personal had done this procedure. Surely it was bad enough she had to endure the stabbing tubes inserted through her back into her pleural chest cavity. Donna reported this procedure was always "fine "or" good." She knew what to do, the routine; gravity draining fluids and sometimes blood for two or three litres at a time. She had palliative radiation on her abdominal mass for ten days at Oshawa Hospital, in August. It had worked! She did not need to have a paracentesis; fluid drained from her abdominal cavity. Her abdomen was not filling up, needing to be drained, as it had so many times before, throughout the past year or two. This symptom was related to her ovarian and abdominal cancer. This symptom was NOT occurring, but was controlled again. A palliative care *Blessing!* We were so thankful that this symptom was gone now.

The home care nurse was with Donna when I entered. I'm foggy now. I can't remember. I did have some catch up time with my brother-in-law outside while the nurse assessed Donna. She was in her Lazy-Boy chair, oxygen humming, trying to focus on what the nurse was asking her. I think I said hello and went outside with Jeff. "Are you OK? Is Mom OK?" "How is

Donna today?" He replied, "I don't know. You think you are prepared for this for years but now, I find I am not." Donna's weak. She had gotten up in the middle of the night to go to the washroom and thank goodness Jeff heard her. He got up to assist her. She was too weak to manage the tubes needing to be organized as she walked. She had been too weak to even shampoo her hair. Not Donna, always pretty.

That afternoon, I tried to encourage Donna to rest after her nurse's assessment and visit. I showed her my YouTube recent videos. One featured my husband Jamie fishing and catching a Northern Pike. Another featured my gardens and humming birds, and one of me, after catching another large Pike. I thought this activity, which required no energy on her part, would take her mind off other things. I nattered about the inconsequential happenings in my life.

Jeff had reviewed the morphine pump and oxygen working details with me and the emergency medication she may need: Ativan. Ativan is a quick acting relaxing medication. I didn't recall, but was reminded later by Jeff of something I said that first time we helped Donna settle into bed together. I had needed her to be still while her lines were organized. I jokingly said, "If you don't do what I say, I won't be your nurse and I'll go back home." Little did I realize that she took this to heart. She would listen to me, respond, cooperate and focus. No matter how distressed she was, she committed to me, even more so now. She remained true to her conviction, showing her determination to respond to my instructions and encourage- ments. No matter how distressed her poor body was at the time!

When I suggested a toasted tomato sandwich for lunch, she had to spring up out of bed and go in the kitchen. She tried to make the sand- wiches, grabbing a bowl, not a plate. Too weak to do this chore, I raced to organize the tubes behind her and to support her at the kitchen counter. I said I'd do it and commanded her to sit down. Her reply was, "I'm sorry but you may not make it the way I like." Of course when her appetite was now so small, wouldn't ensur- ing your food was 'perfect' be a priority? Our family had always loved our food. She instructed me in the kitchen while I took over the sandwich preparation. No butter, minimal mayonnaise, just the way she liked it. Ice in her juice; taken through a straw.

Settled again, she asked me where Jeff was. She had forgotten we told her that he was out doing errands. She would push her 'bolus' button on the morphine pump, which gave her an extra dose of morphine, if prescribed. She fumbled for the buttons.

Donna did rest after this episode of exertion. I couldn't focus on any laptop work. I just sat my chair beside her and watched her, absorbing her condition. She lay in a hospital bed with the head raised, oxygen on, breathing laboured, sallow and pale with her wrist and shoulder bones protruding.

She was scheduled to have her thoracentesis, "lungs drained," on Friday. Her breathing would get worse daily as nature and this disease took its course.

She bolted up again saying she needed to go to the washroom. I helped her get settled there and went to the hallway to allow her some privacy and dignity. Next, I hear her bending over the tub—what the!!! She could fall, injure herself. "I want a bath," she said as she quickly stripped off her clothes, short of breath. I was again torn apart by her unabashed behaviour. It allowed me to see the condition of her poor body. The breast rash, also a form of the cancer was in fact all over her upper torso; red, blue, thick and scaly. Was that actually skin? I tried to show no response, just to react to conserve her energy and give her what she wanted. I got her sitting down with a towel for warmth and ensured the tub filled up at her appropriate temperature.

We had crossed this bridge before, last spring when the tub was her only place to get comfort from pain. While she had sat in her bath tub relaxing, I insisted on sitting on the floor beside her to keep visiting. The curtain pulled slightly to allow for privacy, but both of us relaxed enough to just enjoy our conversations while she enjoyed some comfort.

I put a couple of violet rose bath bubbles in the tub and we watched them swirl and dissolve. They smelt nice. She said I was always so thoughtful. Gracious still in her disease, ridden body and mind! Wow!

She tried to pull herself out of the bath tub with the bar handle, but could not. Confused, she said, "I can always do this, now I can't." Even she could not keep up with the physical changes occurring within her body. Her voice sounded so surprised. Nurse mode "kicked in." I quickly assisted her to sit on the edge of the tub. I then swung her legs around, a lift with her arms around my neck, and she was stable and upright. She was exhausted. I asked her to sit on the toilet seat while I remade her bed, wanting her to rest before the next movement, the long walk back to bed, twenty-five feet or so.

In order for her to feel in self control, in control of her house hold, she asked that I put the new lambs' wool on her bed. I said, "sure thing." Settled again; bolas of morphine; Ativan; with juice through a straw. Exhausted, she slept.

Jeff came home and went to check on her. She roused immediately, but was still groggy. We knew she would rest longer. I told her we were going to sit outside and would peek at her. Her reply was, "Well, I'll peek at you peeking at me." I said, "OK, we'll play peek-a-boo!" She smiled and drifted back to sleep.

"How are you Jeff? How did it go? How was Mom?" I knew Mom needed to talk. Needed comfort after this 'funeral experience,' but Jeff needed it more. He proclaimed, "It was tough, but the administrator at the funeral parlour helped make it easier. Mom did better than I thought she would. It's a beautiful casket with roses embroidered, a matching guest book and even the Urn has rose tapestry on it."

I felt sick at hearing these words, but knew that Jeff needed to talk about this experience, somewhat.

With permission from Donna's doctor, a nurse could now 'pronounce the death.' The family would just need to make a phone call to the Community Care Access Center (C.C.A.C.). This organization would also call the funeral director to take the body to the funeral parlour when it happened. I told Jeff about Donna's sandwich event and the bath earlier today. We went back to "peek" at Donna resting.

"I need our marriage certificate, clothes for her, a picture and a 'funeral poem." Jeff recalled that the marriage licence was in the wedding photo album. We looked for it among her thirty or more other photo albums. My sis loved family pictures. She had them all organized. No wedding album was found. I grabbed two baby albums, one on each of her children. We quickly searched the house and still no wedding album. Panic!

Donna can't die until we find this! Jeff remembered that Erin their daughter, youngest child, had had it out on her last visit. "I'll have to ask her on the next phone call if she knows where it is."

I phoned my mother's house to see how she was. She was visiting and dropping something off at my Step-Aunt Faith's, who also lived in the Victoria Place, V.P. subdivision.

I knew she respected and needed Faith's knowledge and compassion; female compassion; another mother. I have no children and cannot pretend to understand the anguish of losing your first born daughter. Faith is also a knowledgeable career Palliative Care Nurse. She had helped Donna immensely with a couple of urgent situations in the past. Bless her heart. Her family had moved back from the U.S.A. and had forged bonds with ours. I hadn't seen Faith for over twenty years, or was it thirty?

Jeff invited me to supper. Jeff cooked and served grilled chops. He had been doing all the cooking, shopping and household chores for years. Donna was only able to join in on occasion, on a good day. On a bad day, she may have criticized his work, being angry: the stage of dying. Her harsh words about a task done 'improperly,' from her viewpoint, allowed her to still be in control of her household.

After supper, I took Kayla for a walk to the community lakeshore and "doggy" beach. We flushed a grouse on the wooded trail. I let her sniff around at the doggy beach and get a drink from the lake. I needed to gaze at the calming water. I couldn't find the same wooded trail on the way back as late dusk was upon us. The trails were shadowed. Oh well, I took a trail and went out through the neighbour's back yard, then to Donna's house.

Mom and Len were visiting now. Jeff and Len were doing the 'guy thing' in the living room, allowing Mom and Donna privacy while watching "Idol" on TV. Only to me, Donna did not seem comfortable, eyes closing, laboured breathing. Thinking, how come this stupid TV show is on? Her brain cannot absorb this. Direct simple sentences are best, less confusing. It had been Mom and Donna's habit to enjoy a few different TV shows together in the evening. Even in the hospital a few weeks ago, Donna had been anxious to hear the latest happenings on "Idol."

That last hospital stay in August was when they set her up with "The Morphine Pump." She was stronger then. I had now, having this one day with Donna, a better comprehension of Donna's health than my mother, a retired Registered Practical Nurse, R.P.N. who had devoted the last twelve years to helping her first born daughter deal with cancer recurrence and remissions? She had slept in Donna's hospital rooms from Peterborough to Oshawa to Kingston, sometimes weeks at a time. My sister had clung to her mother, Mommy. They shared Florida trips, a cruise and shuffleboard tournaments, not able to turn into the driveway of their own houses without each other knowing; seeing. They lived just three doors away from each other. This was the start of an occasional 'Nursing Conflict,' and the start of the official "Nursing Team."

After about twenty minutes, I said that Donna should go to bed; it's been a long day. Mom looked alarmed. "'Idol' wasn't over and Donna would want to see it all!" "No, she's been up enough." My mother said, "Well, I'm the senior nurse!" I retorted," I'm the up-to-date nurse!" Donna said, "Yes, I'll lie down." Jeff had jumped up, half an ear to the girls happenings, his eye trained on Donna always. We got Donna ready and settled in bed. Mom kissed and tucked her in. I had to get back for 'medicine dog' now. I had Kayla on a later insulin schedule so I could be there for Donna's bedtime routine and so I could sleep in a little later.

Back at Mom's, we talked and cried about the funeral arrangements. We had a few laughs with the snorting dog Daisy and Kayla. I did an email check for my business and had to say goodnight early. I was tired, too much to absorb in 24 hours. Mom mentioned a book left by the C.C.A.C nurses. It was on the bedside table. I wanted to read it and this book was a *Blessing* too! The book became such a useful tool for our family. Condensed wisdom of the stages of dying; it promoted understanding of the dying process; physical changes described. These changes could be expected and watched for. Fears of Donna's health changes could be alleviated with understanding in their place.

5

September 11th, Thursday

I drove over to Donna's again. I was anxious to see how she was today. How was her night?

The home care nurse was there. Donna in her chair, but a bit slumped forward with her head drooping, startling herself into awareness for the nurse's assessment and questions. She was polite and calm in her responses. The nurse spoke with Jeff privately again. What did that mean? Further guidance or is this bad news? Then she left.

Donna and I heard Jeff visiting with neighbours outside. He came in and asked Donna if it was OK for Janice to visit? He knew from past years that when Donna felt sick, she liked the privacy of solitude from friends and associates. She was always "Fine" when in public, fashionably dressed, hair done and make up in order. Would she allow this friend and neighbour to see her? She said OK. A lovely lady, Janice, entered with a beautiful bouquet of flowers. I helped carry on some small talk. When this lady asked, how are you? Donna replied, "Pretty good today." She sat up straight, eyes and mind focusing on the present. Was this the same Donna who was nodding off a few minutes ago? Janice kept her visit short. She had a gracious warm hearted good bye and hug for Donna. She was in tears as soon as she was out the door. Saddened and shocked by Donna's obvious decline and frailty.

To my surprise, Donna spoke clearly saying, "Why won't they stop! The phone has been ringing all day! Can't you make them stop?" The phone had not rung once. Where was Donna's mind? I told her I had taken care of it. "They were not going to call and bother her anymore. Let's get you to bed." With a bolus of morphine; holding her up, aligning oxygen cords and morphine pump pole. In bed she said, "They are saying I am bad, why do they keep phoning here?" "No, they will NOT call anymore. We stopped them," I replied sternly. She laid back her head seeming to try to understand this. Anxiety and troubled fear had shown in her eyes, those gorgeous big eyes of hers.

She grabbed the phone and started fumbling with the keypad, fingers missing the numbers. She knew she couldn't perform this task and that scared her too. "Can you call Mom for me?" I dialed and gave her the phone. I could only hear one side of the conversation and Donna seemed to be relieved, putting her head down. I indicated that I wanted to talk to Mom also and she sighed and closed her eyes. Mom asked, "What's going on? Who's calling?" I replied very quietly, "No one, never happened." Donna was always in tune with what was being said if she wanted to be. I didn't want to upset her.

I went to talk to Jeff. Wow, the energy she exerted with Janice totally played her out! The brain needed to rest and went into its fanciful wanderings. Telemarketers! She hated them. Jeff said she used to blow a whistle in the phone. Childlike, she took her relaxer pill (Ativan) with juice and ice through a straw. She asked if we had any orange juice, as she was tired of apple. She rested, breathing more laboured today.

I asked Jeff, "How was she last night? Did you get any sleep?" Jeff did sleep but it scared him. Things were not as he had left them last night. Donna must have gotten up by herself! He cannot believe he didn't hear her. I offered to take the night shift tonight. To sit with and watch Donna all night; Jeff hadn't slept for days.

My Auntie Marion, Mom's sister and Uncle Gord were expected to arrive today. They did not know I was there. They knew the pressure of Donna's illness was acute. They were coming to support Mom, Jeff and to see Donna. One last time…we all knew it would be her death, soon.

Mom's sister had supported her with grieving my Father's passing. Auntie Marion loved and shared a continuous relationship with Donna, her first niece, her bridal flower girl. They shared the same wedding anniversary date. Donna had arranged her wedding on that day to commemorate and be 'special' for Auntie Marion and Uncle Gord. Their arrival was another *Blessing*. Mom needed this support. I can move into the McCauley household now without alarming Donna. My aunt and uncle can settle into the starry Dungeon spare room.

Word was spreading in this retirement community. Things at the McCauley household were getting tough!

Over supper, brought over from a neighbour, complete with homemade carrot cake, Jeff told me that our nurse had advised him to phone their children and tell them the 'end' was near. This would ease their shock. Let them decide what to do. The kids lived in Kentucky. Another horrific task for Jeff today!

Later that day, My Auntie Marion and Uncle Gord, with Mom and Len, came for a visit. I realized they had spent extra time with Mom before coming to the McCauley's. Mom, no doubt, needed someone to cry with. This would help her deal with the trauma of planning her daughter's funeral arrangements.

I left Donna in Mom's care as she needed 'her private' time with Donna. My Auntie Marion had brought with her a special prayer for Donna. A woman from her church had written it with my Auntie Marion, especially for Donna. My loving aunt was in tears after seeing how Donna had deteriorated, withered to her current ghostly state.

Tea was given to the men in the living room. Awkward times, nothing they could do; as men prefer to do something. Fix the problem. But no one could. We tried to share pleasantries and a semblance of normality. I ended up passing out some magazines I had brought with me. Technology and inventions stuff, perfect for Uncle Gord. I thought this a *Blessing* too. Why had I thrown these magazines into my suitcase?

I asked Uncle Gord if he'd like to go for a walk with Kayla and me. I always enjoy special time with him. We have a connection as he has no daughters. Let the ladies visit and care for Donna for a while. Jeff was always hovering in the background and would be there in a flash if there were any problems.

Donna did have episodes of severe respiratory distress. Anxiety would increase this, making it much worse. She would call for Jeff and he would stare into her eyes and willfully coach her to breathe slowly, rubbing her back soothingly. She always responded to him. He knew what her needs were; when her last bolas was; when she could have Ativan. He knew what her stomach could currently tolerate—ensure (a nutritional drink), ice cream, baby portions. He made a lot of good soups! Jeff was keeping track of when she should rest, best as was possible, as the changes in her condition were now happening quickly. She was weakening daily. Jeff was always there.

Uncle Gord and I enjoyed our walk to the waterside doggy beach. We enjoyed the calming sunset over the water. It was a dark dusk when we found the wrong wooded trail back to the McCauley household. Me, getting lost again! I asked Uncle Gord if they could stay another night. Their intent had been a one-night visit, but we needed them. I couldn't look after both Mom and Donna. Upon our return, Mom and her sister were ready to go home. "You sleep in Donna's room this evening, OK?" Len had brought over an outdoor lounging chair they believed I could put in Donna's room and sleep on. "OK?" Mom insisted. Hugs with all and then Jeff and I are alone.

I gave Jeff some private time with Donna while I showered. With everyone trying to help, he had been denied time with his wife.

Friday, tomorrow, was the dreaded day! Donna had to be in Peterborough at the Catheter Lab to have her lungs drained, thoracentesis. How the heck would we manage that! But if we didn't, the fluid would kill her!

Later that evening, Jeff called his son, David. Being honest, frank and calm, he told his son the situation. He then handed the phone to me. It seemed important that David understood that his mother did not expect either of her children to come and be with her now. She understood and knew the kids had jobs, university and that David and Kathy would be here on September

19th for the engagement party. Kentucky was a fifteen hour drive south. Erin was mothering her three month old baby and tackling a Masters Degree full time. With finances and time tight, she wouldn't be making it for her brother's engagement party.

Donna wanted that 'party' to happen. She enjoyed the phone calls to plan and prepare with her son and fiancée. She was willing herself to hang on for this. But it was only September 10th; would she be too sick to attend? I told David how happy his mother was in knowing he would be getting settled in life, married, starting a family some day, having a new core family in Kentucky; no longer alone in the USA. I told him that's all that matters now. She was not in pain. He is a quiet thoughtful man, my godson, my nephew, thirty years old now. His response was quiet. Did I scare him? What was he thinking? I handed the phone back to Jeff, I think. I can't remember. I do remember questioning Jeff and his response reassured me, "It was good, what you said." He reassured me that it helped.

Jeff hadn't slept well for days, weeks; really it was years, as he supported and loved Donna with her illness. A constant drag on your soul! A heaviness of heart; anxiety, as a way of life for years! Sometimes critical, sometimes calmer states of the disease, but more intense is the emotional turmoil. It was my evening to sit with Donna. Jeff put the coffee pot on for me; considerate even in his state of mind. He asked if I'd like the lawn chair, but I declined as I was too much of a sound sleeper. If Donna woke, I'd never hear her. The bed side chair was fine. Finally alone, Donna and me! I enjoyed my 'nights' with her; our private time that week.

Uncle Gord had surprised me with a book he had researched and found about the St. Mary's River. Our summertime canoe trip to the ship wrecks on the river, near my house, prompted his inquisitive mind to search for and find this book. His love for me prompted him to give it to me. Another small *Blessing!* It was interesting reading material and would keep me awake and entertained while Donna slept.

But all I wanted to do was talk to her, watch her. Her breathing very laboured; head of the bed up. Try this neck pillow—big smile—"It's good." Her forehead un-creased as ease came to her body. She would mumble—awake or not, I don't know. I put my legs up on her bedside and settled on my chair. We looked through both David and Erin's baby albums that night. I would describe the pictures and compliment her on the "amazing Christmas" they had. The floor loaded with presents for the kids, smiling children. Her lips would curl up in a smile with her eyes still closed, a mumble, and, "Yeah we did. I'll be better tomorrow after I get my lungs drained." She was in tune enough to have this appointment, or should I call it an event, imprinted in her mind. Treatment kept her alive. She always wanted treatment no matter what the side effects were. She never actually focussed on any of the pictures. I do believe her mind gave her even better pictures of the loving memories of raising her children.

I kept a constant morphine bolus going. Jeff advised when Ativan could be given. She had asked for her bedtime pills. She knew she was tired, due to company with auntie, uncle, me, etc. I told her I had my computer and would get some stuff done and also would read Uncle Gord's present. "So sleep when you can, so I can start!"

I held her hand all the time. Touch is a comforting sense. I fondled her hair, rubbed the side of her cheek. I put the support pillows in place if she turned and made her comfortable, helped her be peaceful, happy and content. Hopefully dreaming of happier days! She muttered, sometimes clearly, sometimes not.

I remembered how much it meant to me when Jeff told me that Donna asked for me when the phone and doorbell rang. Her confused thoughts were also a vital part of her, and sometimes they were comical, I recalled that 1:00 p.m. phone call Mom had related. "Mom, send Jeff home to make supper!" Donna had implored.

I paid attention to this muttering and jotted down what I could discern:

1. Want me to get the camera for Jeff? Good, she is remembering about 'loving' times?
2. Canada—Is she now living memories of her ten years in Kentucky?
3. Necklace—Well, perhaps she's dressing for a special time.
4. Come sit here (and she patted the bed)—I jumped up and sat where she indicated. 'Oh that's nice.' She smiled with a peaceful expression. She was asleep and would not know I was crying. Some tears fell on her and I thought she wouldn't notice. They kept falling. She asked, "What's leaking?" I told her the only thing I could, "I'm crying. I'm so sad you are sick." "Oh," she said. I leaned down and hugged her. Her arms came up around me, even in her weakness she said, "I love you." "I love you too." I told her how proud she should be to have such wonderful children and family.

Enough! This isn't helping Donna! Or is it? Honesty in sickness? Good or bad? If I was dying, wouldn't I feel better if someone asked me if I was scared? Or told me they were too? Donna hugged me tightly.

I decided that honesty and frankness was definitely what I would give Donna. If you had no one to confide in, you would feel too alone. It would be scary and isolating. She knew she was dying. How and when were the questions—what would happen next? The scary unknown!

I gave her a morphine bolus and Ativan. She slumbered, again in and out of muttering.

5. I can do that…no problem!

I got a bit cocky and thought perhaps I could 'play with her head' and carry a conversation with her in this jumbled state. After all, she was my sister. She knew I could be bratty and teasing. I'm not doing a 'nursing' nightshift. I smiled at the thought. With my legs sharing the bed while I sat in my chair, I held her hand— this is much different.

I said to Donna, "You are dreaming." She replied clearly, "I think you are right!" I chuckled and she slept on.

Now she pulled her hand away and started to stretch them out and grasped, working her fingers together; outstretched them again. She's definitely doing 'something.' I let her work on this project for a while. "What are you making?" She was startled and confused. "I haven't got a clue." I laughed. She settled her head back and entered into an exhausted, medicated sleep again. I just stared at her alot through that night.

I found and read the Community Care Access Centre book on the Three Stages of Dying. I cried. The book was good. Understanding the process of the body's changes took the fear out of these occurrences. These changes would be expected, watched for. My hospital nursing training was recalled. It's been twenty years since I was a 'bedside' nurse. I had been a good one.

I read some of the St. Mary's River book, but couldn't focus on it. I never bothered with the computer; no way would I be able to have the mental focus. Adrenaline was keeping me awake just fine!

Jeff roused and came to the door to check on us once or twice. He's forgotten how to sleep! Always on guard for Donna and any potential needs she had. He was now sitting in the reclin-

ing chair and I went to see him. Pale, sweaty–
"What's up?" Jeff's blood sugar had dropped to
2.1; juice in his hands. Oh no, alarm flew
through me! "Can I get you anything? More
juice? Protein?" I went from patient to patient,
Jeff to Donna. He insisted he was OK and also
insisted that I didn't tell anyone. His blood
sugar level came up to 7. He went back to bed.

6

September 12th, Friday

Morning came: I had to stay awake to give Kayla her insulin and then lay on the downstairs bed for an hour or so.

It was now time to take Donna to the Peterborough hospital for her thoracentesis. But how? I washed up and dressed. I had brought a poncho with me; perhaps it would be handy to help Donna's dignity. She was short of breath. How could she dress? Mom was already in the living room helping her stand and organizing a housecoat around her. Mom announced that she'd have to go like this; it was too much for her laboured breathing and weakened state to dress her.

At the doorway, I thought to ask Auntie Marion if I could have a copy of the prayer she and her friend had written for Donna. She gave this to me with a hug. I put it in my purse at the doorway. This prayer was a wonderful *Blessing!*

Do we have a chair on wheels? She cannot walk alone. Can she make it to the car? We'll help her. No time to argue, no other options. With assistance she made it to the car with the portable oxygen, morphine disconnected. Mom drove; Jeff in the front seat and Donna and I in the back. She was exhausted. I cradled her head and shoulders in a hug. I told her she could sleep all the way there: just like we did as kids coming home from Friday night visits at Auntie Phyllis'. Five cents was given to you if you were awake at the end of the trip. It was years before we were told that our father invented this five cent incentive so he wouldn't have to carry three girls into the house! We usually were roused from sleep just before pulling into the driveway! The lure of five cents gave us the stamina to walk inside to bed.

Mom and Jeff talked just a bit. We were all too stressed to do more than focus on getting there. As I hugged Donna, she would smile and relax as much as her laboured breathing would allow. Her eyes continued to be glossy as she struggled to be alert.

Forty-five minutes later we arrive at the hospital. I eased myself out of the back seat to race for a wheelchair from the foyer. Slight conflict occurred as Mom and I both tried to support and transfer Donna to the wheelchair. Of course, my method was best and I took over. Mom graciously allowed this. Mom parked while Jeff and I wheeled Donna to the elevator. Jeff coordinated all her 'lines' and portable oxygen.

Donna struggled to remain sitting and coherent. Boy, she looked worse when compared to the 'mainstream' of society. So frail; hollows under her large beautiful eyes.

We registered at the Catheter Lab reception desk and Mom appeared. They were expecting Donna so, a quick phone call to the lab and she was on her way. Settled in her stretcher bed, we gave her hugs. Donna said, "It's OK, I'll be better after this."

Mom waited with Donna as I was getting 'burnt out,' tired. I waited with Jeff. We all got Tim Horton's coffee from the small stand. It was a busy line up as the hospital staff was taking their breaks.

Jeff took me past the Palliative Care floor in this new hospital. This was where Donna spent ten days in August. The nurses and doctors were good there. It was set up well. Out the side entrance we went, and down the roadway to the smoking area (off hospital property). A hospital receptionist was there. Of all things, she said she recognized me from my August trip to this place with Donna. Coffee and cigarettes were good; stimulants to keep me awake. Who knows how the procedure was going. Tubes punctured into her pleural cavity! Fluid and blood drained by gravity!

It was good to talk with Jeff. I can't remember what we talked about, but we stayed out there awhile. Nicer, and perhaps easier to wait outside the confines of a depressing hospital waiting room. Mom was waiting for Donna's return and they usually kept her for a while after the procedure to ensure there were no complications.

When we returned to the waiting area, I went on through the 'interior private doors' to find Mom and Donna in the 'step down' room. Mom said, "What took so long? She was done for awhile now!" Oops, we're in trouble, Mom's stressed. I replied, "Sorry, but that was faster than usual. How much did they drain?" I changed the conversation focus. "Has Donna had a good rest after the procedure?" A nurse advised that one litre from the left lung and one and a half litres from the right lung. Fluid and blood had been drained. I said, on more than a couple occasion, I was happy Donna had had her Post Op rest time. She had no chest pain post treatment. Mom was 'wound up.' We focused on getting Donna back into the wheelchair. I asked Donna how it was. She replied, "Good this time," with eyes sleepy and oxygen still on.

Settled again in the car, we returned to our 'hugging' position in the backseat. I think Donna was de-stressed on the drive home. Mom and Jeff conversed more on our trip back to the house. Len was waiting and had taken care of my dog, Kayla in my absence.

With Donna now settled into bed, lines reconnected, I went for a walk with Kayla to the doggy beach. Mom had time with Donna.

I don't remember what we did this evening or what we had for supper. Did I lie down again? As Donna needed some quiet sleep now, Mom and Len left for their home. Everyone was exhausted from this experience.

Jeff advised me that their son, David, was coming up from Kentucky. He hadn't been able to get in touch with their daughter Erin yet. Wow, David was taking time off work and driving up. It was about a fifteen-hour drive from

Bowling Green, Kentucky. What a wonderful son. I excused myself now, as Jeff needed some one-on-one time with Donna.

I took a shower and focused on cleaning up the basement for David's arrival. Jeff came to see what I was up to. I said, "Don't worry, just the white tornado or quicker picker upper!" I was trying to help out with the household chores and would clean up his tea cup before he was even done! But he had set it down in an obscure place, who knew he drank warm or even cool tea! I don't think I got any rest that day. I thought the tidying up for my nephew David was very necessary.

A phone call came later. Jeff said that their daughter Erin and baby Grandson, Wyman are coming too! Wow, imagine these beautiful kids would risk a lot of hardship, organizing work, organizing Masters University and tending to a three month old baby on a fifteen hour drive, all at the last minute. Now I vacuumed and cleaned the upstairs too, as the "baby" would be here.

Before I knew it, it was after 11:30 p.m.! Jeff and I sat outside after checking on Donna. I told Jeff how great the C.C.A.C. book was. I was getting worried that when Erin and David did arrive, their mother's condition would scare them. We decided we needed a bit of 'one on one talk' with 'the kids' to prepare them before they saw their Mom.

No, we were not telling Donna that the kids were on their way. She would worry. It was her time to be surprised. Paybacks! Just like Mom was surprised at my arrival!

The kids also needed to know that when talking with their mom, sentences must be kept simple, clear and short. Otherwise, her mind would get too confused, overwhelmed. I wondered, how do you tell Donna that her children have just driven fifteen hours in an urgent frenzy as they, and everyone else, knew that she would soon die? How do you tell her? Wouldn't that terrify her more? They are coming because you are dying! I thought this and felt like Jeff sensed this in me.

I resumed my bedside position, holding her hand. She'd mutter in her sleep. I remember crying again, praying. I would kneel and pray for guidance. How to help? How to do the right thing for Donna? To help her find Peace! To help her be pain free! To help me help the family! The *Blessing* of our C.C.A.C. Nurse helped us. Jeff said she advised him to just say, "Donna, look who's here to see you, Erin and David." Say no more, no less. Don't complicate things. OK, I felt that we had a plan. Off to bed

Jeff. I wanted my time with my sister, my precious night shift!

I read my Auntie Marion and friends special prayer for Donna.

> *Heavenly Father, You look after us and continually hold us in Your arms. Your strength can carry us through any situation. We lean on You now Lord as we come together and lift Donna up before You. May Your grace light her Life. May Your peace; the peace of God that passes all understanding, saturate Donna's body, mind and spirit. Please surround Donna with Your ever-present angels to comfort and strengthen her. We pray for healing and freedom from pain. And Father, please be with us all and guide us on this journey. In Jesus' name we pray, Amen.*

I did my internet check for business while in the room. It's very important that a dying person remain 'with' the family. Not 'tucked off' in a lonely bedroom, isolated. The computer room was a great place for her. As well, accessing the head and three sides of the hospital bed was important. It was workable here. Only a few days earlier, Donna had been able to watch the photos that our nieces Amanda and Jennifer, had on their 'facebook' pages. The week before, she could reply to email with assistance from Jeff.

Donna always checked and emailed our family which was spread from Ottawa to Whitby to Kentucky to Sault Ste. Marie. She'd email or forward a joke or poem to aunts, children, and friends on a regular basis throughout these last years; a couple of notes a week. If you didn't get a few emails, you assumed she had failed and was back in the hospital. At one time, she was using Internet Access right on her hospital floor!

Jeff peeked in the room around 3:30 a.m. I think he saw me crying. "Come sit outside, tea, or maybe coffee?" I had started to borrow Donna's sweatshirt hoodie for chillier times. It didn't matter if I got it smoky. She would never wear it again...Jeff and I talked. Not so much about Donna, but of Jeff and his interests. His recent information tracing his family tree, his Father's death, and the war medals his Dad would not accept, everyone in war was a hero. Then we talked about Donna and his first date and the special times they had while dating. We talked about some trips they had taken and the weekend outings they enjoyed together in Texas.

We had thought the kids would arrive around 4:30 a.m. or so, but couldn't tell for sure. Driving with a three month old baby would require several stops for breast feeding. So we kept on talking. Jeff had been a brother to me since I was eleven years old. He had so much stress in these past years! He needed someone who knows Donna closely and knows about their history, but also someone that was removed from the day to day intensity. Not mixed up in the 'care giving,' ups and downs, as my mother was. I was a bit of an 'outsider' as I participated with Donna's emotional care mostly by phone and email. I had made four emergency trips to visit and help in the past two years. I know that Jeff mainly shouldered his burden alone! Time did fly by as we talked in between checking in on Donna. We found her muttering but no major upsets. Around 6:30 a.m. or so, the car pulled in the driveway.

It was our turn to run out to the driveway! Erin, my niece, immediately cared for her three month old baby boy Wyman. Poor fellow, strapped in the car seat for all those hours! There were hugs for everyone. My nephew David was such a grown up man, but was made fragile by this tragedy. David was already on his way to Canada, in Ohio, when Erin called on his cell phone. David had turned around and went back to Kentucky to pick up his sister and baby nephew.

Inside now, Erin was changing the baby's diaper. Jeff was saying his hellos and inquiring about their trip. There was commotion with bringing in suitcases, diaper bags and playpen from the car. We all tried to keep it quiet, so not to disturb Donna. Jeff and I told the kids that their Mom did not know they were coming and that we needed to speak with them for a moment before they saw her. A startled stare; then we continued to help organize the playpen and luggage. I carried most of the bags downstairs and allowed Jeff to have private words with his children. I was nervous for Donna, such an overwhelming surprise.

Joining Jeff, we kept our explanations with the kids brief. Jeff told his children that their Mom had gone down hill alot since their last visit. I believe the nurse in me, chimed in and explained that her body was quite frail and that she was on oxygen and a morphine pump all the time to help her. "Don't worry about the lines and cords; they are 'good things.' She is on heavy medication and it's hard for her to focus on long sentences, or quickly changing ideas. At times, her mind wanders. We try to speak simply and directly to her. She'll be so happy to see you both!" Jeff went to Donna to tell her the kids were here.

David looked solemn and pensive. Erin, wide eyed with those same beautiful big eyes as her mother, only glimpses of fear and tears seemed to sneak through her composure. Wyman let out a small cry.

The kids entered her dimly lit room. 'Hi Mom, we came to see you." They moved closer to the bed. Donna sat straight up, her face turned beat red and as her body rocked back and forth, she cried, "I can't believe you are here!" That moment, watching that moment, being a part of that moment, was truly an honour to share. The most intimate, almost sacred part of the McCauley family!

"Baby Wyman, here he is." She repeated through her tears, "Oh baby Wyman, David, Erin, I can't believe you are here!" "I want up," she proclaimed and rushed to swing her legs around. I rushed closer to steady her and organize the lines and pumps. Donna was up and almost bolting for her chair in the sitting/TV area, still red faced and teary.

They talked and I believe baby Wyman was put on her lap. The exertion of tears took a toll on Donna's breathing. She was gasping a bit. Jeff gave her an Ativan. I took this moment to straighten out her bed and give them some privacy. About ten minutes was enough and Donna needed to go back to bed. We said that the kids had been driving and needed to sleep as well. They would all see each other later when everyone was rested.

After Donna was settled back in bed, I had to say it, "So Donna, we managed to surprise you! Just like you kept a secret from Mom and let me surprise her! Pay-backs!" A smile, laugh, "Yeah, OK." She eased back into the pillow, now content.

7

September 13th, Saturday

I can't remember what happened today. I stayed up for Kayla's medicine. Mom was back over. Erin had to stay up to look after Wyman and managed to nap when he did. I remember giving her a bagel. I was outside with David, Uncle Bruce, my step-uncle, and Faith's husband, Jeff, and a couple of neighbourhood men. Mom and Faith were with Donna.

David and I sat on the grass. I needed to read him and Erin the C.C.A.C. book on the three stages of dying. I asked him if I could do that with him now. I wanted them to understand what was happening to their mother and that it was normal; not scary! There was a medical reason for her present state of weakness and I also wanted them to understand what to expect in the future.

As I read the three stages, I'd interject "I'm sure your Mom has this," i.e. depleted oxygen supply, or, "we haven't seen any evidence of that yet." He was attentive as we leaned together on the grass; me quietly reading aloud with David following along. That over with, I interjected in the men's conversation on the porch. I added my two cents worth of nonsense conversation to change the subject, to lighten the load.

I think this was the first day I really talked to Faith. She's a bit more than ten years older than me, so hard to call her aunt; and step-aunt even more ridiculous. "Hello Faith, Hey." She broke the ice by telling me that Mom had told her what strength I had shown these last few days and nights. My Mom was amazed at how I was helping out. I replied by saying that was nice, but I was just doing my part. I remember Faith and Mom talking back and forth to Donna at her bedside. Mom sitting with tears in her sallow eyes. No one had been sleeping well, even if they had an opportunity. Worry was increasing daily, hourly.

I remember Erin changing baby Wyman on the red blanket I had given him spread down on the living room floor.

Kayla got her medicine. Jeff asked for a lesson with this in case I ever needed a hand.

Kayla was good. Jeff would be able to do this if needed. It was so thoughtful of him to request this lesson, especially when he had so much to think about.

People seemed to be everywhere in the house now. The dishwasher always needed to be filled or emptied. Laundry was started, then forgotten, then finished. The two cats, Gump and Starla, needed feeding. Jeff would lose track of time. Together we tried to keep the two pets fed and their litter boxes clean.

David went to bed first. Erin and the baby had more 'minutes' with Donna while she slept, or was vaguely awake. I showered and blow dried my hair. It felt good to be clean, more human.

Later that morning, or had it turned to after-noon, Erin was in the downstairs bedroom with Wyman. I asked her if we could read the C.C.A.C. book together. I told her that David and I had already done this. We sat on the bed together in our own private world of tragedy as I read about the three stages of dying. Sniffle, eyes welling up with unshed tears! We hugged and I teased her about sharing the bedroom with her and the baby's playpen. She needed to breastfeed Wyman. She was exhausted. As she settled in for a feed and hug with beautiful baby Wyman, I left her.

I went upstairs. Mom and Faith were almost 'guarding' Donna. Jeff was on the phone outside talking with his brother. I wanted to call Darlene, our sister, but couldn't find my address book. No one was conveniently around to provide her phone number. I read the prayer Auntie Marion had left in my purse:

Oh heavenly Father. You look over us and continually hold us in Your arms. Your strength can carry us through any situation. We lean on You now Lord as we come together and lift Donna up before You. May your grace light her life. May Your peace, the peace of God that passes all understanding, saturate Donna's body, mind and spirit. Please surround Donna with Your ever present Angels to comfort and strengthen her. We pray for healing and freedom from pain. And Father, please be with us all and guide us on this journey. In Jesus' name we pray, Amen.

I went downstairs and lay on the couch under the quilt Mrs. McCauley, Jeff's mother made. David was in the bed and Erin and Wyman were in the downstairs bedroom. Both kids were educated on the stages of dying. OK, now I was able to sleep for a couple of hours.

Jeff came to attend the litter box downstairs. I said 'Hi' and he was startled, not realizing I was on the couch, under the quilt. He replied, "Denise, you can sleep on my bed in the daytime!" I replied that it was OK; it was time to get up anyway.

I grabbed some fresh clothes and washed up in the downstairs bathroom. Gump the cat was there. Although he was an affectionate pet, he couldn't socialize therefore could not have free roam of the house. He was living in the downstairs laundry room and bathroom area in the fall/winter and outside in the summer. It was difficult to walk around as Gump moved with your every step trying to rub his purring head and body up against you.

I went upstairs. David was at the dining room table in front of his computer laptop. He needed to do some 'work' while he was away. He was an IT, Information Technology Specialist with a company in Kentucky. Oh good, he would be able to help me access the wireless network on my computer. I hadn't been able get it to work on my own laptop and had been using Jeff's PC every night to access my emails and correspondence for our tourist business. He asked me how I was trying to 'log on.' I showed him. In his calm, quiet way, a smile spread on his face, "I think I know what you are doing wrong." He seemed to manipulate the laptop somehow and low and behold, I recognized my high speed homepage. "Wow! How did you do that?" He replied, "See this button on the bottom left of the machine, it turns wireless on! Ha! Ha!"

Oh boy, I had learned how to make and manipulate videos and pictures for my YouTube promotions; but no one ever showed me the on button before. Ha! Erin and Jeff were close by and started laughing as well. We all needed a laugh, good medicine for stress! Of course, as others came to visit, I mentioned this 'blonde moment.' Laughing at yourself was a 'safe topic.' We all needed an occasional laugh to help deal with the intensity of death coming in the household.

Mom and Faith had helped Donna to the washroom. The door was closed. The kids, David and Erin, seemed to shrink back in fear at seeing their mother so weak, pale and fragile. Jeff was called to the washroom. He entered. The door closed again! Minutes later, he quickly left and bolted for the downstairs steps. What was up? He marched upstairs holding Gump the cat and headed for the bathroom. A minute or two later he was heading back downstairs with the cat. Donna had thought Jeff had 'put Gump down' and was all worked up; short of breath and crying. Jeff tried to explain that

Gump was OK and downstairs in the laundry room but Donna would not believe it! My goodness! What next? She couldn't think. She just had to see the cat!

The family had eaten while I slept for a couple of hours. The neighbours, yet again, had brought supper. Bless their hearts. The tea kettle was on constantly. Mom was getting very worn down. At 10:30 p.m., I suggested that she get some rest but she wanted to stay. We cried a bit together and talked. Donna had been getting a regular bolus of morphine for days now. Anytime she woke up and seemed ill at ease. The oxygen and the morphine pump were great. The morphine pump was set to administer regular doses. You could push a button, a bolus, for extra doses. If you pushed the button and she was 'over' the prescribed doctor's order, it didn't give her any. We had the liberty to 'push' for more morphine anytime we felt she needed it and knew no harm could come from this. The Community Care Access Centre Nurse would check the morphine pump daily to gauge how much morphine was given and would call for doctor's orders to increase the doses as warranted medically necessary. When the dose was being infused, it made a high pitched purring sound. Donna had clued into this and called it the 'kitty cat sound." She was very cute in her manners then. We tried to give her as much fluids as she would take, with ice, through a straw, as she liked. Hydration was a priority. Ativan could be given to her for increased shortness of breath and/or agitation. She would cooperate with these meds when we asked her to. Her head of the bed always needed to be raised, which maximised her lung capacity. Even though her lungs had been drained a day ago, this time it didn't seem to give her much relief. She remained with shortness of breath, some gurgling. The neck pillow and other pillows were always positioned around her body to help support and comfort her. The oxygen was constantly on. Her poor nostrils got dry. The nasal canula needed adjusting often as it would dislodge from her nose and go cockeyed.

I told her I was back for our evening shift together. She sat up to look at me, arms outstretched and said, "I love you so much, so much." I bent to hug her, arms around her for support and replied, "I love you so much too." I never forgot the intensity of her gaze as she said these words!

The nursing team, Mom, Faith and I with Jeff our mainstay; were falling into 'report' mode, whenever we saw each other. Nurses pass on any details, called reports when they left their shift. Donna's last Ativan time; last morphine bolus time. Her pulse came into notations as well as it was becoming weaker. Her feet were becoming colder. Pulses were hard to find there. She hadn't really eaten for a few days; a spoonful of yogurt or pudding and a bit of Ensure, a nutritional drink. Food was just extra work for her dying body. She didn't need much nor wanted it; Nature's way of allowing the body to work only for vital organs to survive.

Jeff was in charge of the morning and afternoon meds. Haldol, Effexsor, stomach pills. I don't know what all! It didn't matter. I knew the ones which gave relief and freedom from pain. The others could no longer assist in healing her. But she always tried to take them for Jeff. Night time pills signified bed time. She didn't need to try to focus on anything else but sleep after these meds. Her exhausted body could ease as her mind accepted this ritual.

I sent Mom home and told her I'd be here and call if I needed her. Mom exclaimed, "I promised Donna that I would be with her, at the end." My Mother had dedicated the last five years of her life, as neighbours, waking up and checking on Donna. They went on outings on good days. If Donna didn't need her, then Mom took care of herself by keeping in touch with friends, relatives and her companion Len; taking care of their adopted Dog Daisy. Working in the garden and taking care of her household. If Donna wanted her, she would drop all other plans or ideas in her life to be with her daughter.

My father had passed away seventeen years before. He had a lengthy illness of heart disease. Mom had adjusted to a retired pace and nursed him for years. He was on the heart transplant list for months when he finally needed to go to the emergency room one evening in distress. The nurses and doctor took him to a private room for assessment and would not allow Mom to go in. Five minutes later she was told he had passed on. She never forgave them or herself for not holding Dad's hand or being there for his final moments. It was vital that she be there when Donna passed! "Dad always said he got strength and peace when I held his hand. I should have been there!"

Again, Mom suggested that I sleep on the lounge chair in Donna's room. I could not. I was a sound sleeper. Donna could fall out of bed and I'd still be sleeping, sawing logs. I assured Mom I was OK and that I liked the private nights. I would call her if there were any worries, I promised! She left exhausted.

We were thankful that her friend and companion Len was at home to give her comfort and caring. Len is a wonderful man, adopted into our family, her buddy, tenant and life mate. Mom insisted that there was no romance, but I kept telling her that was a shame. We all need love in our life, hugs and kisses. They were caught holding hands when they thought no one was around. We gave up wondering about their relationship and just accepted it and welcomed his love for our family. His British accent charmed me when he greeted me, "Hello Love."

That night, I went through Donna's wedding album with her. We had found it earlier that day as we needed their marriage certificate held within it. Erin had indeed been able to help find this and Jeff proclaimed, "Of course, it had been in the TV area all along." Now we just needed pictures for the funeral card, a funeral poem and verses for the funeral ceremony, an outfit.

That evening, I went through Donna's wedding album with her; speaking very slowly, talking about each picture. How pretty she was and how handsome Jeff was. Donna was a collector of memories. She had a list of every bridal shower and wedding gift given to her. I chuckled as I read some of this. Donna and

Jeff would be married thirty-five years on October 19th. Some of the wedding presents included $10.00 gifts from people. Signs of the times. Ten dollars was worth a lot more thirty-five years ago.

Exhausted, Erin hadn't been seen for a while. It turns out, she fell asleep, clothes on, lying on the bed downstairs. Her face turned to her baby in the playpen. Wyman slept through the whole night, his first time ever. Did God allow this knowing she was exhausted from the long trip? A *Blessing!* I read the prayer to Donna from Auntie Marion. Or perhaps I read it for me; to help give me strength. I knelt at her bedside and prayed. Lord, please guide me. Help me to do, what needs to be done for Donna and her children, our family, my mother and Jeff. I cried more. Then something made me ask Donna, "Will you be my Angel and try to help me do what is right? In life?" I stared into her face as she slept, just looking at her. The household had been quiet for hours now.

David had slept longer that day, but he was up and down. I had some private time with him and Donna. I explained the lines and morphine pump mechanics. An intelligent man, he wanted to understand this to be able to help and not to fear what was going on with his mother.

Jeff, also exhausted, was trying to look after his household. Keeping the family fed with the help of the neighbours, tiding up, having moments with Donna, but allowing Mom her guarded position. We would steal private time while Jeff and I had our cigarette breaks outside, updating one another on issues. "Its OK, I had talked to both kids about the stages of dying." He had talked to them about the funeral arrangements as they needed to be and feel included. David was searching his knowledge for funeral versus. Erin had started to look for the perfect picture of her mother. We needed to find the perfect outfit for Donna to wear, in her casket. It's awful, but was our reality! Having some of this organized would make things a little easier when it happened, when she did die. It had to be soon, her body couldn't go on much longer. Jeff always set up the coffee machine for me before he allowed himself to rest for the night himself; so considerate.

All this welled up in me, kneeling and praying at her bedside. 'Will you be my Angel and try to stop me from doing the wrong thing?'

The quiet of the household was interrupted. A noise! Had the cat knocked something off a table? Had my dog hit something in her doggy dreams? I walked out of the room to look around. I saw something on the kitchen floor and bent to pick it up, and turned it over. A chill went through me. It was a small plastic and ribboned Angel face! Where had it come from? White and pink, a Cherub with short flipped hair, looking like Donna. I picked it up and went back to her bedside. I had my answer. I had my vow she would be my Angel always. Wow! Overwhelmed, I sat and stared at her. The night hours went on.

I needed to continue dealing with the reality of my life, and checked the business internet correspondence. Done. Then I checked for potential flights that my husband could take from Sault Ste. Marie to Toronto, dates, times, prices. He would want to be here for the service or if I needed his strength. Right now, I had no extra energy to focus on him. I needed to be here on my own: but soon…

Then I thought I could search the internet for funeral poems. Although it wasn't my place to pick the poem, I thought it would be helpful for Jeff and the kids. There was quite a lot online. I read many and wrote down 3 different ones I thought she would like. One was my favourite.

'GOD'S GARDEN'

God looked around his garden
And found an empty place
He then looked down upon the earth
And saw your tired face
He put his arms around you
And lifted you to rest
God's garden must be beautiful
He always takes the best
He knew that you were in pain
He knew that you were suffering
He knew that you would never
Get well on earth again
He saw the road was getting rough
And the hills were hard to climb
So he closed your weary eyelids
And whispered, "Peace be Thine"
It broke our hearts to lose you
But you didn't go alone
For part of us went with you
The day God called you home

—Author Unknown

Donna had always had a 'green thumb.' Beautiful flowers inside and outside. In fact, she's the only person I know who had a poinsettia plant for three years. Mine usually lasted about two weeks or so.

I had gone outside for air around 6:30 a.m. and left a soft doggy stuffed animal in Donna's hand to replace my own. When I returned, I noticed she had snuggled this doggy up closer. Adorable.

8

September 14th, Sunday

Jeff was always the first up. He never really slept but needed the down time to at least try, to relax. I told him about my Angel, showed it to him. It had been on the fridge for years. There was one magnetic circle on the fridge. Wow!

David came upstairs. I wanted to talk to each of the kids as much as I could. I didn't get the chance to see them that often. Erin and Wyman were also up. We shared a standing joke that I would change Wyman's diaper, but I first needed a lesson. Unfortunately for Erin, I always seemed to be handy just as the new diaper was being fastened on, job complete. I did 'poop scoop' Donna's yard once and told Erin I would gladly exchange this job for hers.

Mom came over 'Hi honey, how did it go last night?' We exchanged 'reports.' I told her and the kids about the Angel. It seemed that people didn't know what to say. They just tried to take this 'happening' in and absorb the occurrence.

Mom tried multiple times to get me to go to bed. I did have to stay awake a bit longer to give Kayla her doggy medicine.

The home care nurse arrived. I did not always get involved in this visit, as Jeff was the mainstay of this responsibility. He would relay any new information to me. We had grown into 'shared moments' outside while we shared coffee or tea and our cigarettes. I had run out of cigarettes and Jeff had loaned me a huge bag from the native reserve. Inexpensive, but I could not really enjoy my smoke. We updated each other about Donna, the family, funeral plans, nursing measures, the kid's emotional state, and Mom's emotional state. Jeff was showing signs of wear and tear. He would almost react too quickly and forget things like laundry in the washer. I'd tidy up behind him, as a wife would, and finish things off. That took a bit of my time throughout each day. Kidding around was part of the routine as well. We did share some laughs that week. We both knew each other needed this stress relief, badly needed it. In sharing a story, Jeff said, "I'll slap you upside the head!" I found this a catch phrase and invented occasions to 'slap him upside the head' in a verbal threat! We still carry on this joke months later, via emails and phone calls.

On one occasion Mom had left Donna's bedside and rushed out to the living room, to the laughing family and said, "Can't you guys be quiet. Don't you know she's dying in there? I can't believe you can laugh." Oh boy, let me talk this over with Mom. I told her we needed laughter. We needed to help the family, as well as Donna. It would make it easier for everyone to be natural, feel like they could be themselves, under the stressful circumstances.

I told Mom that I was going to her house to have a bath and sleep for awhile in The Dungeon, a good long while. I left around 11:00. I had only eight hours sleep in the past three days. My head felt numb, my eyes hurt. My brain was brittle and numb. Faith was coming over later and would support Mom. Mom again teary said, "That's good honey, you go." The family was quieter and subdued in the living area. I started a 'give a hug—get a hug' regime with everyone.

I enjoyed some quiet time on Mom's deck. I luxuriated in a bath, snuggled into bed in the Dungeon under the big dipper, took one half of a sleeping tablet, and slept. I knew I was living on adrenaline and caffeine. I was too wired to go to sleep on my own. I needed to sleep quickly, to be stronger for what was yet to happen.

It was 7:00 p.m. or so when I woke. Feeling much better; house still quiet. I called my husband Jamie and told him about the available flights. He objected profusely. "How do you know she's dying, you thought this before." How could he know she's dying?

I didn't need this! This stubborn attitude! I told him I'd keep him posted. "See Ya!"

I went back to Donna's house. She was weaker, colder. My sister Darlene, her husband Wolfgang and daughter Amanda were there. Darlene had brought her famous lasagne and salad. Hugs! She and her husband were unable to get some time off from their jobs. The state of the economic recession of 2008, was affecting their positions. Time off would be severely frowned upon.

There seemed to be people all over the place. I ducked out to get a few things; my own brand of cigarettes and some cat food. Bobcageon was only five minutes away. I remembered to get an engagement card for David and Kathy. Who knew when the next opportunity would arise to get out again?

After picking up the cat food at the grocery store, I sat in the parking lot for ten minutes and just enjoyed 'being away.' I missed one turn on the way back. It was now dark. I drove fifteen minutes or so down a country road, turned around and had to backtrack. What next, more Blonde Luck!

Upon entering the house, the three Reiners, Wolf, Darlene, and Amanda, sat at the table. Where is everyone? Was Erin breastfeeding? Was David napping? Mom was with Donna.

Apparently my Auntie Joan and Uncle John had stopped by for a visit earlier in the day, but it was three days later or so before I knew of this. I had been sleeping at the time.

Mom and I talked in confidence stating she was worried that Darlene hadn't had any one-on-one time with Donna. They were sisters, but not buddies. Each had different life styles. Darlene was shyer, especially with 'emotion.' I suggested we have a three sister private visit.

Darlene and I went in to see our sister. "Hi Donna! It's just us three girls, the Three D's." We were called this, the "Three D's" as we were

growing up—Donna, Darlene and Denise. "Do
you remember that Grampa couldn't remember
our names and called us Shirley?" Donna said
no, but Darlene remembered. Donna said she
wanted to sit up. I helped her up and she stead-
ied and focused into awareness. She had always
tried to rally in front of Darlene and most other
people. We reminisced about being kids; and
trailer traveling; going to Six Foot Bay Camp-
ground; the baseball games and the volleyball
court. We talked of Dad's famous breakfast,
bacon and stewed tomatoes. Darlene said she
would make this for herself every once in a
while even though no one else in her family eats
it. We talked about waterskiing, Donna always
drove the boat for Darlene and I, avid water-ski-
ers...and other stuff. I kept the conversation
going when any 'pregnant pauses' occurred.
Darlene also tried to keep this fond reminiscing
going. Donna would say "oh yeah" and smile.
Ten minutes was more than enough for Donna's
energy. Donna was maxed out and Darlene and
her family needed to head home. Good bye. I
helped Donna lay back.

Amanda, Wolf, and Mom were in the little
room now. I 'felt' for my niece Amanda and
tried to tell her something to the effect that her
Aunt Donna was not in pain; that the illness

and her condition were normal for the last days of this illness. She had tears in her eyes. Days later, she told me I was the only one who could make her cry. "I remember at Pop's funeral, I cried when you talked to me then too!" I didn't know that! I didn't remember. What had I said?

Hugs at the entranceway, "Call us." My sister's family, the Reiners, left.

Mom asked me how it went? I knew she meant, "how did the three sister's visit go?" I told her that Donna sat up and participated in our fond reminiscing. My mother asked, "How can you do that?" I believe she would have rather heard that we spent time asking Donna's forgiveness for every sibling dispute we had ever had. Or perhaps, were we to lament how we loved Donna. I don't really know what she had expected. But she seemed annoyed and anguished about the reminiscing. Mom remained not accepting that Donna would pass soon.

I feel that reminiscing took Donna's mind off the present. Not to focus on her fatigued troubled body, but to help relax in pleasant memories. The pain meds worked better in a relaxed body. I don't believe she was having pain. She would become upset and scared with her episodes of respiratory distress. She was scared to acknowledge that her body was failing her, getting weaker by the hour. Strangely, Donna's mental state seemed more "in tune" now. The obvious confusion didn't seem to be occurring. She seemed to be in a groggy sleep/dream and would vocalize her thoughts. Jeff told me that after I left for my sleep at Mom's house, they heard Donna say "Your brothers and you best get dressed. The wedding is soon." She wasn't talking about David's future wedding; she was talking about 'our wedding.' *A Blessing.* I know this gave great joy to her husband to know the value Donna placed on their wedding. A favourite memory! Donna seemed to be making a conscious effort to be aware and cognizant, or to be sleeping or drifting in a relaxed dreaming state. Donna seems to enjoy reminiscing. It validates your life. It helped unite us as three sisters, the "Three D's."

"I just can't do that with her!" Mom anguished.

The household seemed busy with the activity of the baby, David, Erin, Jeff, Mom and Len on occasion. Next, I remember Mom was telling me that Donna was asking for certain people to come into her room. I stayed in the background, checking the internet, folding laundry, making tea, outside with Jeff, a doggy walk? I don't remember.

As my night shift hours approached and people started to go to bed, I sat with my mother at Donna's bedside. I hadn't been 'called' to her room. She did say to me, "I love you." I said, "You forgot the So Much." She smiled and said whimsically, 'so much, so much, so much, so much,' and lay back down. A smile on her face, her hands stretched upward as if an orchestra conductor, dancing to her whimsy 'so much.'

Mom was hesitant to leave that evening. She knew, as I did, when people say their last loving thoughts, they often allow themselves to sink into a blissful death. We both had this new fear. Was death a bit closer now?

It was about 1:30 a.m. Monday morning, when Donna bolted up. "I have to go to the washroom!" Mom said, "OK honey, we'll help you." It was getting harder to help her walk. Weakness was preventing her strength. Laboured breathing increased dramatically with her every movement. She had such a determined mind. She wasn't going to wait for us to arrange the oxygen and morphine lines. She wanted to move now! Mom and I acted as an efficient nursing team and scrambled to organize her encumbrances. Both of us supporting her, we made it to the washroom with her oxygen and morphine pump. She sat on the toilet. I declared that I was getting Jeff. Mom asked, "What for?" I was scared. Often people feel the urge for the bladder and bowels to release just before they die. Many people do in fact die on the toilet. My mom said that Dad felt this way before she got him to the Emergency Room. I knew Dad had wanted to stay in the bathroom. Mom had called my sister Darlene and her husband Wolf that night. They helped talk Dad into going to Emergency. I woke Jeff and told him this fear. He was up in a heartbeat.

We gave her Valium while she was on the toilet. Jeff rubbed her back and shoulders. "Settle a bit, and then we will help you go back to bed." She listened.

Now 2:30 a.m., Donna settled, exhausted, head up, breathing laboured, but calm. She was getting accustomed to this distress. Her feet and fingers were cold up to the ankles and hands. Her pulse was weak. She wanted Minister Daniel to see her before she died. Jeff declared, "I'm going to call for him."

Erin and David each came sleepily upstairs. Jeff had awakened the kids. We hugged and told them that the minister had been called. We were in and out of Donna's room, holding her hand, touching her cheek; her adult kids, husband, mother and myself. Len was called by Mom to come back over to Donna's house. We made and served coffee, checked on the sleeping baby, Wyman. At last, a car pulled in the driveway. Sarah, the minister's wife, got out. She was also a minister. They work together at the local church. Quick hellos and introductions were made to all. Extra chairs were put in Donna's room. The lights dimmed.

Earlier that day, Mom and Faith had started playing soft music in her room; a wonderful calming thing for Donna. She had a series of gospel CDs that she loved to listen to. She often listened to them while she was living in Texas. Her best friend in Texas was the minister's wife. This evolved friendship was a *Blessing* as her religious faith was renewed then. It had helped her immensely when she received her terminal diagnosis five years earlier.

Everyone crowded in her room. There wasn't much space left. Mom patted the bedside and told me to jump upon the bed and sit there. I did. Sarah read passages from the Bible. The atmosphere was surreal; hymn music in the background; all of us listening and focusing on Donna. She would twitch, her mouth often twitching into a smile. I thought she's reaching out to the heavens, smiling. "Yea though I walk through the shadow of death, I fear no evil, thy rod and staff they protect me…" This was the only passage I remembered, the only passage I recognized. All the words were comforting.

Sarah's voice was soft and soothing. Erin was solemn, sad with tears welling up in her eyes. Mom was panicky, alert, on edge, hyped. David was comforted, absorbing the scene. Jeff was solid, watching all. Len held Mom's hand. We were all tense. Donna continued to reach up musically; not responding to us but seemingly aware of Sarah's words. Smiling! Then Sarah shut her Bible and was done. I went with my instincts and read the prayer given to me from Auntie Marion.

Oh heavenly Father, You look after us and continuously hold us in Your arms. Your strength can carry us through any situation. We lean on You now Lord as we come together and lift Donna up before You now. May Your grace light her life. May Your peace, the peace of God that passes all understanding, saturate Donna's body, mind and soul. Please surround Donna with Your ever present Angels to comfort and strengthen her. We pray for healing and freedom from pain. And Father, please be with us all and guide us on this journey. In Jesus' name we pray, Amen.

A pregnant pause…then I said, "We make our mistakes in this world so we are ready for the next."

Everyone knew Donna wanted to enjoy and be a beautiful person. But, she also had a grumpy side to her personality. She needed to be forgiven for this. It was my way of explaining this to the kids.

Mom, Jeff, and I went to say our goodbyes to Sarah. She sat with my mother in the living room, comforting her. Even she was aware Mom was the most anguished due to her struggle with acceptance. We knew Donna could NOT continue life in this weakened, diseased body. Mom has focussed on Donna and her health for so long, so many years. She only wanted Donna to stay with us. All logical thinking did not matter. She did not want her daughter to die!

Mom, David, and Erin were sitting in the room with Donna now. Jeff and I took our coffee outside, dawn having shown its dim light. We needed a stress relief with our unhealthy habit, a cigarette. A dark cloud was on the horizon; then a small rainbow appeared. "Wow, that's Donna's rainbow taking her to heaven!" Jeff was amazed. We never get rainbows here. Typically, the weather patterns bring clouds and rainbows over the lake…the opposite side of the house he explained. There was no apparent rain. What a *Blessing!*

Erin walked by after checking the baby. "Look! Come see your mother's rainbow, how beautiful!" We watched as Donna's rainbow faded, peacefully dissolving into the morning sky.

We went back immediately to check on Donna. Was she still OK? Yes, relief!

"When Jeff and I were outside; we saw a rainbow, Donna's rainbow to heaven." Amazement and smiles on our faces! David sharply gazed at us, "We thought Mom was talking about her gardens. She started talking about different colours!" Silence! No one could believe what we were hearing—Amazement! We all looked at Donna sleeping. Nothing could be said about this *Blessing.* It was too great!

I thought that while she was smiling and twitching her hands up to the heavens, she had indeed been on a short trip to the heavens. God wanted her. He had just told her this and He had shown her it would be beautiful; nothing to fear; the glorious beauty of the rainbow. It wasn't necessary for any of us to comment. We all just thought. The baby cried and Erin ran to him.

9

September 15th, Monday

We tried to resume normal life with breakfast. I was waiting for the medicine dog time. There was lots of hugging. David needed to check in via computer with work. The morning nurse would be here soon.

I spoke privately with Jeff. "Can you ask if we could have a night nurse? I'm getting too tired to stay awake. I'd like to sleep with Donna and have the night nurse watch over us both. I'd be there for anything!" "OK," Jeff agreed. We were all showing signs of exhaustion. Faith had generated this idea by telling me in her Palliative Care nursing, when people slept with a patient, they did better. Having perched on Donna's bed, while the minister was there, reassured me it was comforting, and comfortable for Donna. I was too tired to 'be there' for the night shift, any other way.

I was washing up when Mom came to the bathroom door. I quickly asked if Donna was OK. "Yeah, but I think Jeff is upset with me."

The nurse had come and she asked if we would like Donna to have a catheter. This tube into Donna's bladder, attached to a pouch would eliminate trips to the washroom for Donna. She would not use a bedpan, we had tried this already! Mom stated that Donna always got infections when she had catheters. She had to tell them that! Jeff reacted sternly to her as he wanted Donna to have one. She was too weak to get up now! He had snapped at Mom. I hugged my Mom.

I could envision the episode. I could see both viewpoints, but I agreed with my brother-in-law. None-the-less, I did not want to 'side' with anyone. Mom was emotionally frail and exhausted, seventy-five years old. The issue wasn't just about the catheter. It was the bigger issue that needed to be addressed. Who had the ultimate responsibility for Donna's care? Her husband? Or her mother? Differences were established as Donna's illness progressed these past five, indeed twelve years.

Donna valued and took life on with gusto when she remised from breast cancer twelve years earlier. She enjoyed her family, friends, children, work, and trips with her husband while striving to be healthy. She walked regularly, golfed, and participating at TOPS weight loss club. When she was diagnosed as terminal five years ago, while living in Texas, she had needed her Mom, Mommy.

I learned later why my sister had almost flunked kindergarten. She had apparently kept pretending to be ill. The school would need to call Mom to come get her. Instead of allowing the teacher to help Donna integrate and socialize, as the other children were, my mother would soothingly take Donna home and spoil her! Her first born child! So Donna seemed to "play" from husband's to mother's comfort as her illness progressed. Of course, mother thought she always knew best. I told my Mom that Jeff and Donna have been married almost thirty-five years. Jeff has educated himself to the disease process. Donna was too weak for the washroom, too weak to get up, she needed that catheter. There is no way her poor body could last long enough to worry about a simple bladder infection. Jeff was right and Jeff is who the nurse needed to listen to. I told my Mom, "I think you did him a giant favour by being the one person he could snap at. He is also exhausted, stressed and wired. Can't you see that? He can't even remember where he sat his tea cup down! He needed to release this tension. He wouldn't snap at his children, coming all the way from Kentucky. He wouldn't snap at me or Faith. In a sense, we were outsiders coming to help. You are the most familiar. You only hurt the ones you love Mom. Just forget about it and be glad he could snap at you." Mom calmed. We hugged and cried. The nurse put Donna in an adult diaper. Tomorrow we would ask for the catheter.

She will die before the seven or eight days needed for a common, simple bladder infection to take effect. "Mom, there is no way she can last that long, I'm amazed she made it to today!" We went upstairs to join the others.

Erin and David would each be found talking on the phone to their partners. David getting comfort from his fiancée Kathy, keeping her updated, and still arranging for the engagement party which was to be that Saturday, it was Monday now. Brian, Erin's partner and baby Wyman's father was making arrangements to have time off work to come up from Kentucky to be with Erin and the family. Due to the distance apart we lived, I had not yet met Brian. The two of them had visited Donna and Jeff, and Nan, Mom previously. I had seen pictures. Happy smiles full of love for each other. I knew Brian had a good sense of humour. He reportedly called Erin a 'Nan Fan.' Both of Donna's children were especially close to their Grandmother 'Nan.'

Jeff told me that Brian was on his way today. He was expected to arrive around 5:00 a.m. Erin had asked him to come when she realized her mother was 'so bad.' She needed him.

Mom needed rest and went back to her home to shower and lie down for a few minutes. She insisted that we call her if there were any changes.

Jeff and David went to the funeral parlour. They needed to drop off the marriage certificate.

Earlier, I had sat outside with David and he asked me my thoughts on organizing food and décor for the engagement party scheduled for Saturday. It had been planned over a month ago. His future in-laws, fiancée and her brother were to arrive Friday. We looked at pamphlets and discussed food trays. We talked about seating and table arrangements to promote interaction. We thought of decorations and I suggested a quick trip to the Dollar Store. I also suggested that we utilize the beautiful garden flowers from both Mom's and Donna's yard. It was September already and the flowers would not last much longer anyway. It would also be less expensive and add elegance. I was honoured that my Godchild would single out my advice. He knew that I was used to organizing from my lodge experiences.

People were starting to comment daily on what a strong person I was; how good a help for Donna and for the household. It felt weird! I was just trying to keep track of everyone's emotional state and basics of life. Meals, laundry, cats being fed, and Donna's meds, morphine bolus, Ativan routines. Just help. Mom was too old for the night duties. Jeff's health and responsibilities to Donna and his children would not allow him to do a 24 hour duty. I was, in a sense, filling in for Donna. David thought I was good at looking after everyone because of my experience with the lodges. He hit the nail on the head. I was a nurse, but also had been hostess to communities of fishermen at remote fly-in fishing lodges. Taking care of the guests' and staffs' well-being and physical comforts was part of my daily duties there. This boy, now young man, was very intuitive. We would hug and give each other comfort. He had the best 'bear hug.' He was also sensitive. He needed 'special moments' where an older female could give him a chance to take comfort. He no longer had a mother to do this for him. His grandmother could not do this for him anymore, as she was engrossed with her own turmoil over her daughter's illness. Not accepting the eminent death.

I found myself the sole caregiver in the household. Everyone was gone now. Erin was resting with baby Wyman downstairs.

We had a new member of the nursing team coming tonight. I looked at Donna's room and started cleaning; dusting the computer and desk, taping up cards, and arranging flowers for her viewpoint. Donna's hymns or a guitar instrumental CD was playing softly in the background.

Most often the hymn "In the Garden" was playing. A year later, my Auntie Joan shared with me a memory. She and her mother felt they did not have singing voices. Her mother, Nana Ashworth, could be caught singing only one song in the privacy of her home, while doing her housework. She would sing. "In The Garden" Auntie Joan said, "I know all the words!" I too now know all the words. Was late Nana trying to comfort Donna? Another *Blessing* I think.

The music played as I was on a mission to 'spruce up' Donna's room. Donna hadn't been able to do her housework for quite some time now. Jeff had been doing most of the chores. Sorry for being biased here, but he did "Guy Cleaning.' I cleaned the bathrooms both upstairs and downstairs and vacuumed the living room. As Brian was coming, Donna would want this.

She roused once and sat up crying, "I didn't think I would see today, oh why can't I die!"

I climbed on her bed and hugged her exhausted frail body. "Well Donna, I don't know why you didn't die. Perhaps we need to pray and we will be shown the reason for you still being here today. Please Lord, show us your wisdom." I cried with Donna. Again, this moment will be replayed in my mind forever, the anguish in her face, the fact she could confide in me these deepest thoughts. She needed a confidant. She could not approach subjects like this with her children or husband. She would not cause them the pain. But this was her reality, and especially, being a woman, she needed to 'talk' these thoughts. The praying and hugging gave Donna a diversion. She had a strong faith, so found peace and seemed to relax. She entered sleep once more with help from the bolus of morphine and the soothing kitty cat sound.

I was pleased with the household tasks I accomplished. The house started to fill up again. Faith and Mom were back. Faith volunteered to insert the catheter. She was a capable Registered Nurse, but we didn't have the equipment. Mom had resolved the conflict she had with Jeff earlier and now felt guilty for intervening.

A neighbour dropped by with a Sheppard's pie, salad and dessert for the family. Apparently, the neighbours had formed a group to coordinate our meals. Wow, what a community! I also realized that while Jeff was having cigarettes outside, his neighbours would come over to visit with him. Paul and Ron were a mainstay for Jeff's sanity. Nice men and great buddies! Jeff needed to talk about fishing. This gave his mind the stress relief needed in order to continue to live with this terrible progressive terminal disease.

I showered and took Kayla for a walk to the doggy beach. She was behaving so well. Everyone enjoyed keeping watch over her when she lay outside on the soft grass. She had also made friends with the neighbours' Yellow Lab. When inside, she had found a safe place on the dining room carpet to sleep, no one would trip over her there.

Occasionally, when Erin left the soft baby blanket on the floor after changing Wyman, Kayla found it a nice, preferred place to lie. Was it the softness of the blanket or the baby smell that attracted her to this 'bad habit'? Gentle Lab instinct had always made her fascinated with babies and young toddlers.

Faith and Mom were back standing guard. Faith agreed and assessed Donna to be failing more now. Her pulse is thready, weak and irregular. She would not respond to us very often. Some gurgling was becoming apparent with her laboured breathing. "I'm worried," Faith confided. I know Donna sought the comfort of the minister, Daniel. We even had to laugh, Donna didn't die last night as the 'wrong' minister came! "I'm going to talk to Jeff, then call the church and request that Daniel come visit Donna," Faith announced. We all wanted to give Donna exactly what she wanted and needed for a peaceful death. She called and Daniel would come.

A car pulled into the driveway; The minister? No, out came two old white haired people; our

Auntie Joan and Uncle John; such sweet people. Donna had been very close to them, the
closest thing to a daughter my aunt had. "You
know we don't usually just drop in, but we were
so anxious about Donna and thought we could
bring you all supper." My aunt had made Sheppard's pie. We now had two for supper. We
chuckled. Donna had always kept a close eye on
these relatives. When travelling, she always
ensured they arrived at their destination safely.

Uncle John, originally from Holland, was
openly weeping. "It's just so sad to see her like
this. How is she today?" They were told of the
minister's visit, Sarah, coming last night and
that Minister Daniel was on his way. I was surprised to see my uncle so openly crying at the
foot of Donna's bed, not abashed to show emotions. Tears are a way to cleanse the soul, a
healthy outlet for sadness. Auntie Joan seemed
able to converse and be strong for them both.
My aunt and uncle were active in the religious
faith of our family, church goers, every Sunday.
Was it a *Blessing,* that they were drawn to visit
Donna now with the minister on his way? I
thought so…maybe this is why she did not die
last evening.

Minister Daniel arrived. Introductions were
made. The family crowded into Donna's room.

Daniel sat and read from his bible, melodic, soft and soothing. He'd flip pages and continue on. The joys of the afterlife and heavens were talked of. He continued this for twenty minutes or so. Again, Donna seemed to twitch with a smile and occasionally reach up with her arms. I stood to Daniel's right, allowing my niece to be in front, caressing her mother's shoulder. Watching everyone, solemn, tears, wide eyed, Auntie Joan, Uncle John, Faith, Mom, David, Erin, Len, Jeff, and me. Donna lay with eyes closed, oxygen humming. When Daniel stopped, the 'pregnant pause' of silence returned. I repeated my aunt's prayer.

Oh heavenly Father, You look after us and continuously hold us in Your arms. Your strength can carry us through any situation. We lean on You now Lord as we come together and lift Donna up before You now. May Your grace light her life. May Your peace, the peace of God that passes all understanding, saturate Donna's body, mind and soul. Please surround Donna with Your ever present Angels to comfort and strengthen her. We pray for healing and freedom from pain. And Father, please be with us all and guide us on this journey. In Jesus' name we pray, Amen.

I believe I said a little more. I don't exactly remember exactly what else I said.

Minister Daniel got up and we followed him into the living room. Between Mom, Faith, Jeff and I, someone was always with Donna. The minister joined us for supper. He spoke graciously with Mom and Faith as he detected their need for his comfort.

My mother told me that the minister had asked if I was 'of the Ministry.' "Oh my gosh! You've got to be kidding!" No one had ever thought that of me before. I was somewhat intimidated by 'formal religion.' This freaked me out!

Uncle John hugged me repeatedly saying he never knew I was so spiritual. This freaked me out too! I busied, checking on Donna, preparing the dinner table and the Sheppard's pie. Faith was an awesome help in the kitchen as well. We would laugh over the extra preparations, like finding the 'good napkins.' We reassured each other that this was a good meal for all, including the minister. Faith said she considered herself a 'country bumpkin.' I told her that was great and that's why we got along so well, because I'm really just a 'northern bushwhacker.'

Faith had been focusing on Donna's condition and assessment. She was a 'mainstay' for my mother; A rock. Caring and consoling as only another mother could be. We also had stolen conversations to update each other on the household's emotional status. I soaked up her palliative care knowledge. She was the one who told me of the extra comfort patients received when they slept with someone. She solidified my idea to sleep with Donna tonight. There had been no time to sleep today. In fact, when was the last time I slept? Sometime through the course of those days, I teasingly said she could be a 'surrogate sister' to me. She was too young to be my 'Step-Aunt' and perhaps I felt too old to be 'niece.' We were related and both outsiders trying to fill in the gaps and bring peace to Donna and her immediate family.

Dinner was had. All was nice. Daniel the minister left. Auntie Joan and Uncle John left saying they would pray and come back anytime. Please let us know...tears.

Mom was now approaching exhaustion. No one had slept much. I believe Len talked Mom into going home. We assured her we would call if anything changed and reminded her that she was only three minutes away.

I wanted to give Jeff and the kids more private time with Donna. I retreated downstairs to clean some more before Brian's expected arrival.

I was cleaning the bathroom when Erin shouted, "Aunt Denise, come quick!" She had run downstairs to get me. "What's up?" I said, bolting for the stairs. "Mom wants to get up to go to the bathroom and we can't stop her!"

I ran upstairs and into "Donna's room" to find her naked at the side of the bed, face reddened with anguish. "Oh why won't you let me go to the washroom? I have to go!" she pleaded. Jeff hovered over her trying to reason with her. She was not strong enough. She insisted she had to go and why wouldn't we let her! I tried to stare into my sister's eyes, willing her to focus on me while I helped support her back and shoulders. The pump and oxygen cords were tangled between her arms and legs. I said, "Donna, you can lie back down and we will put the diaper back on so you can go." She replied, "Oh no! I need to go to the bathroom now!" Tears were in her eyes, face reddened. I reasoned that if she had some how found the strength to sit up at the bedside and take off her clothes, then her determined mind would settle for nothing else but for us to help her walk to the washroom. She was too much a lady to use the diaper. I proclaimed we'd take her to the washroom, but told her to wait until we organized the 'cords'!

Jeff supported her while I untangled the lines from her legs. I think we both supported her under the arms and said, "OK, let's go!" Her willpower gave her extra strength. There were tears in her eyes. We supported and half carried her to the bathroom. I think she was still naked. Time was of critical essence to her.

Erin was transfixed in the doorway watching this scene. The cancerous scaly red blue rash on her mother's chest and torso was an ugly sight. Oh no! Donna had insisted that none of the kids, or anyone other than Jeff, Mom and I, would witness this ugly head of cancer revealing itself. This was too personal for Donna. She had apparently downplayed this symptom. Jeff later confided that she had indeed been living with this cancerous reminder for years. She had told me about these symptoms only months before and said it had progressed quickly. Did she say this to me in order to prepare me for these days of nursing care?

The gurgling in her chest and hyperventilating she was experiencing, were at their worst! Oh please Lord, don't let her die like this. We heard her 'tinkle' in the toilet; such a small amount. This had caused so much upset! Jeff was trying to sooth and support her while she was sitting on the toilet. We had shut the door to the bathroom. I ran to get her some Ativan and juice. She took this as she was told. I then ran to get her some pyjamas.

"Keep breathing Donna! It will settle down soon. It will be fine soon. Just stay with Jeff here until its better. A few more minutes should make a difference." She was focussing on remaining in control of her breathing, of her life. We waited. In, out, in, out, we coached. Donna's breathing slowly started to settle as she slumped into Jeff's support.

Now, how are we going to get her back into bed? She is really too weak now. We didn't have much time to waste. She needed to lie down now. I told Jeff that I would teach David the 'fireman's' lift and we would carry her back to bed. I left the bathroom to see Erin huddled beside David. Together seeking comfort in each other on the couch. Tears were in Erin's eyes. I explained to David that we needed his help. His mother was too weak to walk and that he needed to learn the 'fireman's' lift. "OK," he was immediately attentive. "Let me see your hands. We position them like this." I grabbed my forearm above the wrist. "You do the same. Our hands and wrists form to make a chair. Your Dad will manage the lines. Ready?" We went into the bathroom. Donnas was too weak to boost herself up on our chair. The three of us wiggled around the toilet and morphine pump. David and I leaned down to Donna to make our chair. Jeff boosted her up and somehow managed to transfer Donna. With the pyjamas secured, Donna sitting on our chair, we straighten up. This was much harder on my back and legs than I had thought it would be! I braced myself and willed for the strength to stand up. Donna seemed to loom up high above us. We needed to keep her relaxed so her breathing would remain stabilized. I said, "Now Donna, we are going to give you a Princess Ride back to your room. Pretend you are on a ferris wheel, just like that first date with Jeff." The four of us moved through the bathroom, hallway and into the bedroom. Donna seemed to smile and enjoy her Princess treatment. Perhaps the extra Ativan had settled Donna into this moment, and the distress of five minutes ago seemed to be forgotten. She was a heavy, 'dead weight.' Jeff laughed at the 'Princess' comment. His laugh helped us all ease into a more relaxed mood. He has a wonderful laugh and Donna responded with a smile. We made it to the bedside with Donna now sitting on my lap. "Easy now, Jeff will fix your 'cords' then we'll get you all the way into bed, Princess." I squeezed my way out from under her. We boosted her into bed with her head up, exhausted now and sleepy. The oxygen was back on, bolus of morphine given with its kitty cat sound. Jeff was at her bedside.

"Thank you David, you were wonderful! A great fireman!" Hugs with him too; tears in his eyes. "Oh yeah, I'd count on you in any rescue situation. What a team. Thank you." I needed to praise to make their memories of this experience positive. I went in the living room to see poor Erin alone, horrified and crying. This is another memory I will never forget. I approached her and held her face in my hands, ensuring she looked directly into my eyes. Ensuring she would understand. Calmly and purposely I said, "It's OK. There is nothing that can happen that we cannot handle, Nothing, OK?!" She hugged me.

I was downstairs later that evening when Erin came out of the bedroom. She had been crying. What would I be thinking and feeling if I was her? "Are you afraid this will happen to you?" She leaned into me in a hug.

"Oh Honey, I can promise you, this will never happened to you! We are smarter than that now! I vow I will always keep you informed and protected from this, this Genetic Predisposition! It will Never happen to you…or any other relative of ours! We're smarter than that now! OK?!"

She sniffled, we hugged. I loved her so much. My sister, Donna, used to tell her daughter, "You're just like your Aunt Denise!" I loved this, but indeed Erin has a depth of character all her own! Perhaps being more of her mother's daughter then even she realises!

I had to continue running upstairs to complete my task…

Donna slept. I think Jeff and I de-stressed outside. Erin and David helped each other de-stress. Quiet now. About 10:30.

Jeff was OK with Mom's intervention regarding the catheter. I relegated to him the conversation I had with Mom. Both he and Mom calmed shortly after the incident. Mom was just being a Mom. She now realized that Jeff needed and wanted her input. She learned to ask him for a private moment to voice her concerns. He was a devoted husband and would consider and want all input, but he did ultimately hold the final responsibility for Donna's healthcare decisions. He had Power of Attorney, but more important, Donna had given that responsibility to him with trust and love. Mom now accepted this. I was miffed, upset and frustrated with the episode. I needed to vent, and did so with Jeff in private.

"Those poor kids! Scared to death! Poor Donna!" She has always been particular about personal grooming and hygiene.

My sister's strength of character was indeed impressing me. One time in conversation she said, "You're the strongest person I know." I told her I wasn't, that there was always room for improvement. My adventurous spirit had fooled her; my struggles as a young adult. Donna was proving to possess inner strength and willpower beyond my wildest dreams, far beyond my expectations.

I know I'm getting mixed up with events now...it's a month later. We still grieve, trying to heal. It bothers me a lot that this most important event in my life is now a jumble of memories.

I can now understand why a Palliative Care doctor had advised me, "A Death is like a Birth." An intimate close personal life changing event—one happy, one sad, but both emotionally impacting, intimate; 'The Ultimate Experiences.' I have no children by choice. This is my 'Ultimate Experience.' I must have this journal. I must give myself the peace of mind with the knowledge that I will always be able to recall this time. As I age, as time fades our memories, I must know that Donna's death can always be recalled. It is too important to forget!

Perhaps Mom came back to Jeff's later that night. Or did the catheter incident occur on Sunday? I'm not sure. I don't want to ask Jeff or Mom. Everyone is dealing with their grief in their own way. I don't want to upset anyone with my personal need for this documentation, so I'll continue to assume Mom returned to Donna's after a rest.

I know Jeff and I were in the driveway when the night shift nurse arrived. We spent some time updating her on Donna's weakness and on the family dynamics of who was in the household. I felt such an instant like for this nurse; tall, blonde, trim, middle aged, with a big smile. She assessed the household and the bedroom set up. She asked Jeff for applesauce or pudding. We had started having difficulties giving Donna her meds. Donna was willing, but her body was not responding as well. She could no longer suck fluid from her straw very well. This nurse showed me how to crush the Ativan and mix it with applesauce. One spoonful was easier for Donna to swallow on command. She also prepared an extra apple medication mixture to have handy, just in case. She moved the oxygen machine into the bathroom, quieter for the family, and easier for the 'lines.' I touched base with Jeff. He had a good feeling about this professional caregiver too. Great, because I was so tired! I needed to sleep but also needed to be with Donna. My night shift, my trouble shooting of 'unknown' problems, Donna responding to me. I couldn't leave her alone at night. My obligation; I had made it my own.

I knew I was focusing on staying awake. Critical moments were fine. The body and mind respond. Completing tasks like the household tidy up were fine. But I could feel a haze taking over my mind when I did not have a specific purpose to focus on. I was consciously spacing my caffeine intake and fresh air to help me stay awake.

As this nurse, was in fact a Health Care Aide, she was not qualified to press for more bolus morphine. I assured her she could rouse me to do this, at least every two hours or sooner if Donna showed any distress. I told her about the 'kitty cat' sound being a comfort. She liked that. "I'll remember that for other patients." We talked a bit about generalities. She also worked at a nursing home and had four girls at home. I needed to feel comfortable enough with this person to indeed be able to sleep with her watching. She positioned her chair in the door-way with the hallway light on. I put on the soft instrumental guitar music. If the hymns are playing, I'd only listen to the words and not be able to sleep. I washed up, put P.J.'s on and got ready for bed.

"Donna, this is our night nurse. She's going to help us out tonight because I'm too tired to stay awake. You'd really like her. She's tall and blonde and kind of like me." She was. We enjoyed the *Blessing* of another miracle in hav-ing this health care aide that seemed to 'fit in' with us; our family; Donna; me. "I thought I'd curl up in bed with you Donna and our aide will keep an eye on us both!" Donna smiled and said, "That's nice. That's good."

Now, how was I going to do this? A single hospital bed provided by the Community Care Access Centre, Donna's lines, and the head of the bed elevated for Donna's breathing made climbing in bed precarious. We assessed that if I slid in the left side, put a pillow to soften the bedrails, then I could spoon Donna and make us both comfortable. Spooning is curling up side by side, my front to Donna's back. I slipped my left arm under her neck. Her poor feet and shoulders felt cool, bony, where there once was a supple body. We had been positioning Donna with the support of many pillows. Bedsores, the breakdown of flesh with the pressure of the body and bed were a hazard. Shifting the bodies position from side to side with pillows at her back, buttocks, feet, between her leg; was all very important. Donna eased into my embrace, "That's nice." "Now you go to sleep so I can too." "OK, I love you," she murmured softly. Our night nurse asked me if I was comfortable and added another pillow at my legs to soften the pressure from the side rails. "Oh, thank you for tucking me into bed also." I closed my eyes. Instead of worry for Donna, I felt only her warm comforting body and the peace of knowing I could indeed sleep. I was there for any unforeseen happening. My foggy mind eased into blissful sleep.

Mom must have come back to sleep on the couch that night. I remember the next night she did for sure. She told me that next day she had talked to our aide, reflecting what a beautiful thing it was to see her two daughters hugging and sleeping together. She took a picture. Donna seemed to 'rest' more peacefully that night. Rest more soundly. Feeling safe; being hugged.

I woke about 2 a.m. Damn!! I needed to go to the washroom, bladder pressure! Donna was sleeping calmly. OK. I saw the chair in the hall-way with our health care aide sitting, head slumped down, book in her lap. Was she sleeping? Dozed off? Resting her eyes? I quietly slithered my arm from under Donna and crawled down to the foot of the bed and out. Our aide didn't move. Oh no! I know this poor worker had two jobs. She could very well have fallen asleep. She's only human! She could get in serious trouble for this. The ultimate sin for a night worker! She would feel very humbled and uncomfortable with our family if I was to make an issue of this. I didn't think she deserved this. We all 'maxed' ourselves out sometimes. Who knew what was going on in her personal life or why she was so tired as to 'let this happen.' We had just asked for a night nurse that morning. Perhaps her personal schedule and other job obligations hadn't allowed for her to have a nap before the night shift. I needed to walk by her to get to the washroom. Her chair was blocking the door. I put my hand on her upper leg, rubbed it a bit and said, "I need to go to the washroom, sorry." She instantly moved her chair and I passed. I took my time in the wash-room to give this woman a chance to 'get her bearings' from the sleep that I had presumed had overtaken her. I was personally mortified that our 'night watch' nurse may have been asleep, but now she would also know that she had fallen asleep and was probably also mortified. I reasoned that she would be extra conscious to NOT have this occur again. She would likely be transfixed on us now. No good would be done by chastising this woman now. I slipped back into the room. Donna was sleeping well. I adjusted her bolus morphine, kitty cat purr. The household was quiet. I eased Donna back into my arms and went back to sleep. Besides, I was so tired!

Brian, Erin's partner, was due to arrive between 5:00 and 7:00 a.m. that morning. I assumed I'd be awakened with the household commotion, but I wasn't. I had slept. I awoke with the aide's gentle hand on my shoulders. "I'll need to leave in about twenty minutes." I had asked that I be woken to resume watch on Donna and to let the rest of the household remain sleeping.

Mom was sleeping on the couch. She stirred hearing me in the washroom and putting the coffee on. "I can't believe this is happening!" she cried. It was heartbreaking. We hugged, talked and cried together. Our night aide had left. Brian had arrived earlier she had relayed. A blonde woman met him and they went downstairs. Erin, my niece, being the blonde woman she had seen.

Donna had slept so peacefully. She had not stirred and did not receive her extra bolus of morphine as she did not need it!

10

September 16th, Tuesday

I had had about five or six hours of sleep that night. Wonderful sleep! The downside of this was that my body refused to wake up! I felt groggy and hazy. I craved more sleep. But Mom had needed to talk. Shortly after, Mom had insisted I lay down but I needed to stay awake for Kayla's insulin, medicine time.

The household slowly awakened. I had coffee outside with Jeff.

Erin had chosen a picture for the funeral card; her Mom on the deck with bright red geraniums blooming in the flower boxes. The kids all agreed that the 'God's Garden' poem was very appropriate. David had chosen some bible verses for the funeral service.

Mom and Jeff had consulted with each other, and agreed that Donna would wear the outfit that her daughter Erin had given her. The outfit had been bought for a family picture. Donna was so pleased that David had organized a family picture to be taken about a year ago. Erin had coordinated everyone's outfit so they would match, blending colours nicely; Donna wearing a beautiful blue and black blouse and Erin in a blue and white dress.

A tall lanky fellow appeared upstairs, Brian, Erin's partner. Introductions were made. What a difficult way for him to meet the family. What a sweetheart he must be for driving fifteen hours, taking time off work, which they could ill afford. Doing so to support his loved ones, Erin and baby Wyman. He played with the baby while cooing and laughing. Love glowed in Erin's eyes. I had a few moments alone with Brian while sitting outside. I asked about the birth of his son, Wyman. He enthusiastically reviewed this miracle with me. In fact, I learned more details from him than I had heard from my niece Erin. He spoke of Erin with compassion and a deep understanding. I told him he could call me Aunt Denise as I wanted him to feel accepted and comfortable. I told him that within five minutes of talking with him, I had an instant like for him. I did. I had an instant comfort to be with him and instant relief that he was the most suitable partner for my beloved niece Erin. He was a genuine person with a genuine love for Erin and their son Wyman.

It was a nice September. The flowers were still blooming. As neighbours walked by, they said hello, offered to help with anything and inquired how things were. We would reply, "She's peaceful, but time is ending." Some of these people had tears and hugs for Jeff. Although I had just met some of them, the community had heard that I was a 'player' in this vigil, and offered tears and hugs to me as well. With sunshine and mild temperatures and a beautiful view of the lake, how could the world look so nice when Donna's world was so devastating?

The day nurse arrived and I was asked to help insert the catheter. We went into the room and had privacy for this. During this routine, I needed to help support Donna's limp legs so the catheter insertion could be painless and sterile. Donna knew this nurse and relaxed with her. She was very groggy, but she understood what was happening. She had dealt with catheters many times before during previous hospital stays. The nurse advised me of the doctor's increased morphine dose. Donna was getting frequent regular doses. We discussed what, and how much Ativan and Haldol, another "relaxer" medication added, Donna had now needed. This was getting more difficult to discern as Donna had her family nursing team of Mom, Faith and I, and her mainstay Jeff all looking after her. We were all giving her meds throughout a 24 hour period. I decided to make a flow chart of administered medications to document the times Donna had needed her Ativan. A Nursing 'report' was no longer safe enough.

Increased respirations and restless agitated moments; at the first sign of any distress, we gave her help to relax. Relax, feel peace, spending time with her assorted family members. Although we had intense moments, Donna just received more and more *Blessings!*

Erin, Wyman, and Brian left to go shopping for a black dress for the funeral. This was a needed practicality which would help Erin feel prepared for her Mother's death and get her out of the household. Getting away...from the intensity of Death is a necessary survival technique for coping families; a very necessary thing for everyone. Whether it be going to sit on the porch outside, or for me, a dog walk to the doggy beach for solitude. We all needed a break from the stress, the intensity, in order to continue to be strong enough to help Donna. Most of all, Erin and Brian needed time with each other.

David was constantly talking on the phone with his fiancée, Kathy. Ensuring her family trip to V.P. was being organized appropriately. Kathy was setting up the funeral card with the picture and 'God's Garden' poem on her home computer. She has a degree in graphic design. She would also be sending it to the printers. She needed to be included, involved; Donna's future daughter-in-law. Donna had loved her on sight. I hadn't met Kathy, but had spoken with her on the phone once, regarding our cottage advertising. Again, Kathy's values for family, love, sharing and participation showed through in her willingness and enthusiasm to help our family.

Mom went back to her house to have a bath and rest, a break. She said she was OK but I knew she had not had a good rest the night before. She was the one who kept me up since 6:30 a.m. Talking!

I had things to do. I made a chart for the meds. Faith came over and we shared our knowledge. Mom had told her earlier of being accused of being the 'out of date' nurse. Boy did Faith laugh! Seriously, she too was worried about Mom. She confirmed my belief that Mom remains wanting to 'hang on' to Donna. Donna could never get well. Faith knew too that Mom could never forgive us if she wasn't with Donna when she died.

Donna had an episode of severe respiratory distress that morning. Bolting to a sitting position she said, "Oh Why can't I just die!" I replied, "I guess we need to pray again and see what comes next." She had earned her peace with dealing with this disease, cancer. She deserved to relax at death—having it her way, so to speak.

Over a morning cigarette with Jeff, he was the most important to touch base with, the mainstay for his family, an idea formed in my head. I was relegating how peaceful Donna had been while sleeping with me. I asked Jeff if he would like to spend some time in bed with his wife? His head shot up to look at me with a big smile, and his eyes glowed. Then it vanished into concern. "Don't you think I'd hurt her? What if I touch the wrong spot?" I assured him that he would not hurt her as she was on so much morphine. The warmth and support of his body would be so much more comforting for Donna. She would love it! He wanted to, later in the day. In my first private moment with Donna, I told her,

"Ever since I slept with you, everyone wants to sleep with you! Is that OK?" She replied, "Good, Yeah."

Faith had been sitting with Donna, caring for her. We had washed and changed Donna earlier into her favourite navy, paisley silk pyjamas. I knew she felt good in them. We combed her hair and put cream on her dry, cracking lips. The oxygen nasal canula dried the nose. Some non-petroleum cream was applied. I even gave her teeth a good brush with an electric toothbrush. This was a bit disturbing for her limp body and mind. My sister was a dental and orthodontist assistant. She welcomed this. Her poor mouth lining had thickened and there were dry patches caused from mouth breathing due to her respiratory distress. Her lungs were filling up constantly.

I had tried to call my sister, Darlene. She would want to know the end was closer. Her phone line was busy and then I got distracted.

Faith came to me with alarm in her step and in her eyes. Donna's pulses were very irregular and thready. "I think Mama Bear should be here, in the household, just in case!" Mama Bear was Faith's nickname for Mom and a good one it was! A Mama Bear protects her young ferociously!!

I told Faith my idea for Jeff and Donna to nap together. She loved it. Faith proclaimed she would walk over to Mom's and tell the Mama Bear to come back over. She would talk to her in person so Mom wouldn't be as disturbed by the news Donna was failing even more. Faith left for Mom's house.

Immediately I closed Donna's bedroom door, as Jeff was standing at bedside. "OK, get in your shorts and hop in with Donna!" "What?" he replied. "I'm not stripping Denise!" I stated that Donna and he had certainly cuddled as close as possible on the couch when they were dating and pretending to watch TV! I told him I'd be outside. He wanted me to stay in the room, just in case and asked, "How do I do this?" I guided him into sliding in bed beside her. With his arms and his cheek embracing her, spooning her body. Donna loved it! I turned my chair around to face the doorway and pretended to read. Of course I snuck a peak at them; just as I had from the end of my bed as a little girl, as they kissed goodnight while dating. Jeff was whispering in her ear. It was beautiful. He didn't see me looking as he was engrossed in the moment with his loving wife. Oh boy!

My camera is right there on the desktop. Snap. Snap. He didn't know I did this until nine months later. He still has not wanted to see these pictures. I was so happy he had these moments. And happy she had them too. Wow! To be witness to this! Overwhelming! Blessings!

The door opened suddenly. Mom was frantic. "Where is she? How is she? Let me see!" Faith trailed in. "I told her to relax, but she dropped everything and bolted for the door." Indeed, my mother was the Mama Bear! Jeff was shaken into getting up and told Mom that everything was fine. "Here, you lie with Donna while I do an errand. I will be back soon! So come in!" My mom replied, "Oh yes, Donna always liked sleeping with me." In the past my sister had slept in Mom's orthopaedic bed, insisting that Mom slept there too. The rising of the head of the orthopaedic bed, provided so much relief to Donna's lungs as she had battled multiple episodes of thoracentesis and paracentesis. Donna did always manage her symptoms well. She endured discomfort to certain degrees and then conceded to treatment only when she knew she could no longer wait. She fought amazingly!

Mom did remember to tell me she had called my sister Darlene. In fact, she had been talking to Darlene exactly when I was trying to reach her too! Darlene was immediately on her way to join us.

Mom and Donna had a nice nap together, a couple of hours. I had to 'pay-back' Mom by taking pictures of her and Donna also.

To me, while Donna appeared pale and frail, she also had a beauty about her. I told her this. "You're sick but so beautiful Donna." Was this also a *Blessing* or miracle? It reminded me of the inner glow that pregnant women have.

I might have showered or gone for a doggy walk to the beach, or helped organize today's feast from the neighbours. Again, I can't remember.

Our sister Darlene arrived. Hugs! Donna's respirations were laboured, close to Cheyenne-Stroke Breathing. I don't believe she spoke again! The body conserves its blood flow to the inner torso, the organs that keep us alive. In doing this, mucous goes into the throat and the swallowing ability decreases. Breathing is louder and laboured, named Cheyenne-Stroke Breathing, a precursor to death. Her extremities were cold, hands, feet and lower legs. Her pulse remained weak, thready and irregular, but she remained with us.

I had a need to ensure that my sister Darlene also understood the 'Stages of Dying.' That she understood where Donna was and that she was not fearful of the occurrences of Donna's condition, which were natural. We sat with Donna, I closed the door then read the C.C.A.C. book to her. I briefed her on the medication administration chart and our spoonfuls of mixed applesauce and medications. We had prepared spoons organized with Haldol and others with Ativan: the medications we needed to give her for increased distress. When we needed to give them; there was no time to waste.

Darlene took over ensuring that the family was fed and the meal was cleaned up. This came naturally to her, along with her quiet, competent nature.

The household was exhausted, emotionally and physically, Jeff, the kids, Mom and Len. As people started to go to bed, I became more and more anxious. Donna was too sick for me to lie with her now. Our night aide would be back, but she had dozed off last night! I couldn't rely on her to wake me. What was I going to do? Now the family had grown quite accustomed to me being 'in charge' at night.

I went to see Jeff as he went to his room. "Jeff, I can't do this!" I sat on the edge of the bed and cried. "What? What?" he said and hugged me, "It's OK." "I cannot stay awake.

I'm too tired. She's so sick and what if the night nurse falls asleep again!" I started bawling my eyes out. I'm a good crier. My 'wits' were gone, long gone. I will never know if this woman did in fact fall asleep…She may not have…in my frazzled state of mind, had I jumped to a conclusion?

Mom must have been with the kids or Wyman. I think. I knew I didn't want her to know I was breaking down. Jeff and I went outside on the porch chairs to talk. Darlene immediately came to check on us. I was weepy and told them both my concerns. I knew my body could not stay awake. I could not be responsible for Donna. Darlene took charge of me. She asked when I had eaten last? I couldn't remember. She fed me and hugged me. We three formulated a new plan together.

We would set up the lounge chair in Donna's room and I would sleep on this. Jeff would advise the night nurse of our deep concerns for Donna's condition and ensure she knew how anxious we were. This would have to work.

Our same aide came. We introduced Darlene teasingly advising that she was not another nurse! She would be the 'brains' of our nursing team and was recording the medication administration times. I couldn't see straight to do this!

The last thing Donna needed was yet another nurse on the family team!

We settled the lounge chair into Donna's room. The head was raised so as soon as I opened my eyes I faced Donna. I didn't know how Jeff explained our concern to our aide. Whatever he said, he had gotten the message across to this woman. She was sitting at the head of the bed, holding and stroking Donna's hand. The T.L.C., tender loving care, she was giving Donna was exceptional. I now trusted her.

Darlene was trying to sleep on the lazy boy chair and Mom was on the couch. Kayla was on the dining room floor. Jeff was resting in the bedroom. David, Erin, Bryan and Wyman were settled downstairs. A quiet household; except for the hum of the oxygen and the raspy sound of Donna struggling to breath. We had quiet instrumental guitar music softly playing for Donna and I.

I woke up numerous times that night. Whenever my eyes opened, Donna and our health care aide were nestled head to head. She was stroking Donna's hair, holding her hand and stroking her cheek. I believe Donna liked this. She would know she was being cared for with kindness. She would be secure.

11

September 17th, Wednesday

I took over the vigil when our aide left at 7:00 a.m. Darlene made the family some pancakes. People were in and out of Donna's room, including the baby! So this is how Donna had been 'spending her days.' Everyone coming, sitting, talking to her, touching her, talking with each other, sharing hugs, tears and laughs with each other.

Faith and Uncle Bruce were back. I gave the nursing report to Mom and Faith.

Darlene, Jeff and I bonded as we had back in their Dating Days! Thus, some mischief was schemed. While Jeff spoke with the morning nurse, Darlene somehow found a 3cc syringe amongst the nursing supplies. Faith had wanted one yesterday. The applesauce meds were now also getting hard for Donna to swallow, especially as she was not cognisant in her salivary responses now, another 'Stage of Death.' She had no real strength to command her body to move. We needed an emergency apple juice with crushed Ativan in a hollow syringe with no needle tip. I'm sure we could have just asked the nurse for one, but at the time, this was 'the plan.' It worked! If we pushed the liquid into Donna's throat she did not have to swallow. We had every possible emergency planned for!

The day nurse assessed Donna's condition, her morphine pump status and our medication chart. She had contacted the physician and received orders to increase the morphine pump to yet more frequent automatic doses. Donna was being heavily medicated for distress now.

The household seemed busy. Uncle Bruce stayed mainly outside. The neighbours were checking in briefly. People were in and out.

Donna was washed by her three nurses. We needed to cut her PJ bottoms for ease of application. I picked out Donna's favourite pink silk pyjamas and cut the bottoms. Mom got tears in her eyes as this was another reality. Cut the P.J.'s, as Donna wouldn't need them much longer. I wanted her in her best today!

When talking to David, I suggested he pick a special flower from her garden for his mother. She had always prided on her plant called the Flower of David. He brought some to her. The beautiful white flowers filled her room with a mellow fragrance. I had hoped this would allow David to have a singular special moment with his mother that day. I know again, Donna loved it! *Blessings!* David, my Godson, needed extra compassion!

Erin, Brian and Wyman were now a support for each other. The baby was a beautiful *Blessing.*

I showered and decided I needed to lie down. Jeff said I could rest on their bed and I'd be handy if I was needed. It was adjacent to Donna's 'computer room.' Gonzo! Sleep. Blissful sleep!

It seemed I was just enjoying my groggy state when someone touched me and suggested I get up. "Is everything OK?" I was assured it was. I groggily got up and went outside for a coffee and smoke. There were always a few people now on the porch chairs. The neighbour's dog and my dog Kayla had become friends. Kayla had found her favourite patch of grass and seemed to enjoy some attention and affection from all. She never strayed.

Today when I went outside, Kayla had chosen to lie up against the brick wall under Donna's window. What did this mean? Animals are known for their intuitive instincts. Was she intuitive? I remembered Starla, the upstairs' cat, had spent quite a bit of time this past week under Donna's bed, but she never attempted to jump up on the bed or disturb anything. The weather today was nice and sunny. Feeling less groggy and just a bit more awake, I went to Donna's room. Mom, Faith, and Donna's best friend Ann were at her bedside. Tears were rolling down Ann's usually smiling face. Since the three of them were on one side of the bed, I decided to jump back on 'my side' of Donna's bed and lay with her there. Len offered to bring me another coffee. "Perfect, I'll take one, thanks." I had to lie down.

Mom had called Ann and asked her if she would like to visit with Donna, as time was drawing near. Ann had a cold virus and hadn't been over, this last week as she feared she would compromise Donna's health. Ann and Donna had been confidants for each other, walking buddies, doing crafts, exercising, swimming, and supporting each other. True friends!

It was later that day when Mom confided in me that Ann had lovingly explained that Donna had confided she was fearful that "Mom wouldn't let her die." Donna would feel that she was letting Mom down, feel guilty for dying.

Donna indeed had known she would need to die as her body was betraying her mind. She had thought things through more than I realized. Mom tearfully told me that she had told Donna that afternoon that it "Was OK for her to die." She knew and understood that Donna needed to hear this. Mom had given Donna a wonderful gift with these words to her eldest daughter. She had given Donna her *Blessing!*

Abruptly, Donna bolted to a sitting position and struggled for breath. Panic and fear were in her eyes. She couldn't catch her breath. Beside her, I looked into her terrified eyes. I held her arms up over her head. This would help increase her lung capacity. Sternly, I told Donna that "It was OK. The air will keep coming. In, out, slow down, the air is coming, it's OK!" She continued to hyperventilate. I glanced at Mom and Ann while Mom was supporting Donna's back. I reasoned that I had no choice. I couldn't let my sister die in a fit of distress! I assured her that "It was OK! The air is coming and will keep coming. You are not going to die this way!" I had tears in my eyes as I said this. These moments will be another life long memory for me.

Tears were streaming down Ann's face, fear in her eyes. I gave Donna the emergency 'liquid Ativan' with the syringe. Recognition showed in Donna's eyes. The fear seemed to lessen. She trusted my words. Trusting me more than any other human being had ever done before. She flopped back down. Her breathing quieted to its laboured Cheyenne stroke. She closed her eyes. Ann voiced amazement as she exclaimed that I was coaching Donna. I was! I knew Donna could understand. Although she hadn't spoken for a day, she could hear. The last sense to go was hearing. Ann left with Mom seeing her to the door; hugs; tears.

Months later, Jeff told me Donna's last words. She had heard baby Wyman crying and said, "Poor Baby." Jeff had put Wyman beside her on the bed and he settled.

A car pulled into the driveway. Auntie Joan with Uncle John had come. They entered Donna's room. Tears were in both their eyes. Uncle John again openly weeping, exclaiming he couldn't believe this was happening. He praised me for 'Doing what I was doing' for Donna, for the family, over and over again. He used his term of endearment for me "Niece." Again, telling me that I was Spiritual. I really was not comfortable with this as I was only being me. I was praying every minute of the day for God to help me; help Donna; help the family.

I remained lying beside Donna. I was too tired to do more. I watched as different people came into the room. It seemed a constant stream. Mom was glued in her 'Mama Bear' position. Faith, Jeff, the kids and the baby were all trying to support Mom, Nan in her heartache.

It was around 5:00 p.m. There was much commotion in the household. I believe that Darlene and Faith organized supper for all: David, Len, Brian, Erin, Wyman, Jeff, Bruce, Auntie Joan, Uncle John, and themselves—a full house for sure. I offered to watch Donna while everyone ate.

The room was finally quieted. It was just Donna and me. I laid back, head down beside Donna and closed my eyes. They hurt. I had to say this to Donna, and after this, I could say no more. I needed to tell her, be sure she knew. "Oh, Donna, in caring for you this last week, you have given the family so much! We have forged a bond that can never be taken away. In caring for you, we have learned about each other and drawn on each others strengths. We shared an experience which can never be forgotten nor taken away, and will make us a stronger family. Together! You have brought us all together. You have done so much for the family. Thank you. I love you." My vision was blurry with tears. With my head on the bed, staring at Donna, I spoke quietly to her. My arm was still around her neck to support her left arm above her head, to make it easier to breath. The strain in her forehead seemed to lessen. Her big beautiful eyes shined for an instant.

Then as her cheeks twitched in a smile, her chest did not rise. Did she miss a breath? My head bolted up to fix on her face. I strained to clear the tears in my eyes and focused. Another pause, then a breath, she was dying now! Jeff was at the doorway. "Get Mom! Get Mom Now!" Had Erin just entered the room? I couldn't look as I was focused on Donna's calm face, watching her lips and chest. Yes, I'm sure she stopped breathing and the pauses were getting longer. It happened five or six times.

Mom was now in the room crying over Donna's chest, holding her other hand, in a desperate hug. My niece was now in my field of site as I looked up at Donna's face. Erin's blue eyes welled in tears too. I grabbed her hand and held it against the side of Donna's cheek. We were all one. Donna's lips moved as if to kiss all good-bye when the small amount of air left as her lungs had expelled. Then, no more pauses. I saw no more soft gasps. I turned my arm, which was supporting her wrist, to feel her pulse. Three minutes of no pulse was required to pronounce death.

Mom wept while holding Donna. Her face was almost buried in kissing Donna's hand and hugging her. I did not move my other hand as Erin and I caressed Donna's cheek. I did not need to. No one needed to know that I was checking Donna's pulse. I could see the watch that I had borrowed early from Len. Another *Blessing!* He had lent me his watch! In my tired haze, the watch's large face was easier to read than mine. It was later that I learned that Jeff had been standing at the end of the bed, watching over her always, his woman, his wife.

"She's gone." She had no pulse for three minutes. 5:20 p.m.

It was over. I was done. Donna was content: Loved. I knew she had again played a part forever in our family love. She had died 'her way,' a very good way. Thanks be to God.

Part III: Blessings Just Keep Happening!

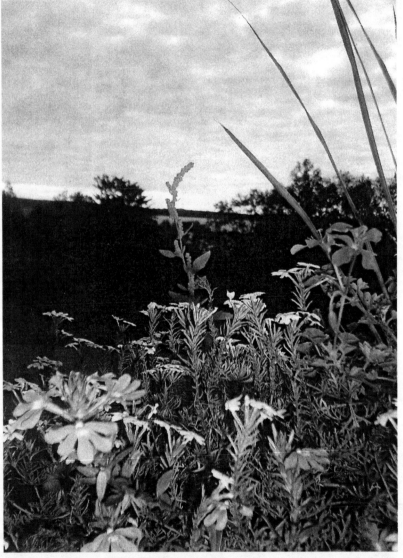

The morning after she passed—the glorious sunrise.

12

September 17th, Wednesday

I got up quickly as others came into the room; Darlene, Faith, Auntie Joan. I left and sat on the soft grass in the front yard. I called Kayla from her post below Donna's window. I hugged my dog.

Uncle Bruce was in the yard. I told him, "it must be like the 'garden poem.' Perhaps God just takes the ones that are ready. The rest of us are not yet good enough." Uncle Bruce was still tortured over losing his younger brother years earlier. His best buddy. He paced in the front yard.

Brian was now kneeling beside me asking if I was OK. What a doll he was to check on me. I assured him I was really fine and just wanted some alone time. I told him I was taking Kayla to the doggy beach and would be back soon.

I walked briskly down the back yard through the solace of the trees. The dog ambled beside me. We passed people at their docks leading their normal lives while my sister had just died. I didn't want to risk saying hello as was the neighbourly custom. I could break down in tears. I kept a good pace to reach the solitude of the doggy beach. I stared at the shining waters of Pigeon Lake, glorious in the late afternoon splendour. I sat down and had a smoke. The dog drank water. I took some deep breaths; in a haze. A minute seemed like eternity. I must get back. Starting home, I thought of Ann sitting at home wondering how Donna was and how we were all doing. I decided to walk to her house then go home. Walking up the hill, the exertion brought me further back into awareness.

I reached her door and rang. Ann was there. I let her know that the Donna had just passed very peacefully. She thanked me: tears. I told her I needed to get back to the house but wanted to let her know. I thanked her for caring for my big sister and being a good friend: Hugs. I had just realized that I had been walking around in my track pants, tee shirt, and, oh no, no undies! These were my P.J.'s from the night before! I laughed! I told Ann this secret. "Don't worry about it! You look fine!" Ann's hearty laugh helped us both.

My attire was all black. Did I wear black to prepare for the grief of this day?

Upon entering the McCauley household, I was greeted with, 'Are you OK?' I started hugging everyone within my reach. I would just have to start 'getting a hug, giving a hug.' David gave me strength with his bear hug!

Mom raced tearfully to me rambling on about how she had prayed and asked Donna to take her with her. What was this? Alarm and awareness shook my tired brain. How could my mother have done this? How could she tell me, her Youngest Daughter, that she wants to join Donna in death! No, I was having none of this! Mom could NOT think this way. If this is her first reaction to Donna's passing, it must not continue. I snapped! "Thanks a lot! After how I tried to help this last week, you are telling me that you want to leave us too? Thanks a lot. Is that what your two living Daughters mean to you? Your Grandchildren? I will not accept this Mom! Stop it! Thanks a lot!" I shook myself and went away.

Faith consoled me by telling me that Mom was just tormented now and not thinking. It was a natural reaction for her: a mother's reaction. I knew that, but was not going to allow her to continue. She needed to be shocked into feeling for others at this time.

I wanted to find the 'kids'. Darlene, Faith, Auntie Joan, Uncle John, Bruce, Len and Jeff were in and out of the house, and her room. Erin was holding the baby in the chair on the balcony deck, outside. Brian and David were there too. Pigeon Lake waters shone with the glowing September sun. Donna's flower boxes were generously in bloom. We all hugged each other. I asked if I could hold baby Wyman; soft and pink, baby skin, baby smell, baby warmth. I looked at my watch. "It's been an hour since your Mother died and here I am holding a miracle of God's giving. Holding this beautiful baby!" A *Blessing!*

Faith and I washed Donna and removed the lines, tubes and catheter. We dressed her in a lacy peignoir set. I combed her hair, smoothed lavender skin lotion on her face and hands; got carried away and applied a touch of pink lipstick. We made a beautiful memorial on the beside table; candles, her flowers from David, her Hail Mary card, my rosary, a cat mug, etc. The family wanted to see Donna again without the tubes and cords.

The family visited, but I avoided this. I had no room left to help anymore. I had said all that I needed to. We saw Auntie Joan and Uncle John to their car. Uncle John lamented, "If you have to die, this was the way to go." Beautifully. Peacefully. Surrounded by family.The Garden Hymn was playing in the background. She radiated in the candlelight. She again looked beautiful. I took another secret picture.

A new nurse came and officially pronounced Donna's death. We had done his job in washing the body; but it was four hours after her death before he arrived. The family hadn't wanted to wait. Faith and I felt that we had done a better job anyway, with love. The old fashioned way. Family tending to Family. My surrogate sister, Faith, leading the way!

I had flashback memories later about trying to close Donna's eyelids. I remembered a phone conversation we had only weeks before. The C.C.A.C. nurse had requested that Donna read the stages of dying book. She had been wrought with tears saying, "Did you know that someone has to close the eyelids?" Of course I knew, but didn't know I would end up being that someone.

Everyone started to go outside. Some were on the upper deck outside and a group was below with me on the lawn. It was dusk; evening falling;

stars were out. We talked about the stars and inconsequential things. I now realized why everyone had left the house. The funeral home had arrived to take Donna 'away.' They also took the hospital bed. This was a helpful thing, but everyone left the house as this was a noisy task. Painful in the thought that was brought to everyone's mind: Moving Donna's body away! Finality!

The funeral home attendants had the utmost poise. Respectful with decorum; but the task was too painful for all. Later, Brian lamented Erin, Wyman and he had been in the bedroom downstairs and unfortunately, the noise was most evident there. What painful memories for Erin. My heart broke, yet again!

I asked David before he went to bed, if it was alright if I checked on him later? He said he had called Kathy and talked at length with her. And "Yes, it would be OK."

I called my husband Jamie. He was ready and would drive to Victoria Place tomorrow. His packing and organizing was done. "But where were his black shoes?" I told him and he found them while on the portable phone. A ten hour drive: "OK, see you tomorrow, be careful, I'm fine, I love you."

Darlene stayed at Mom's house that night. I gave Len instructions on how to take an Ativan before going to bed. "Would he try to also get one into Mom?!" They both needed some sleep. Len was also quietly exhausted and anguished with grief. Darlene took charge and I was so thankful. Everyone was exhausted: slowly seeking their own solitude and rest.

I checked on my Godson and Nephew David. I kissed his cheek, told him I loved him. He was seemingly asleep.

I was alone upstairs with Jeff. I went to my car and brought out four coolers, which I had purchased on my trip down, eight days earlier. No occasion for a summer drink had arisen. In my mind, now was certainly a good time. I orchestrated a private memory to Donna for him and me. I put the song 'Oh Donna' on the tape deck. We toasted. I started with a hug, then a few steps of a slow dance. We sat and listened. 'Oh Donna, Oh Donna, Oh Donna. Now that you're gone, I'll never be the same. How I loved that girl. Oh Donna was her name. Where can she be!' The Richie Valee tune lamented our feelings for us. Jeff downed his cooler in record time! He rarely drank as it could upset his blood sugar. I think I drank two. Tired, and now numb, we kissed and hugged goodnight. It was over now. I cuddled up on the couch for blissful sleep.

13

September 18th, Thursday

We took pictures of the morning sunrise; glorious pinks shining into the sky. I told David that I would treasure these pictures, the beautiful morning. The sky was a testament from Donna to tell us she was at Peace. She was in a better Place. Her *Blessing* to us!

I made pancakes for the family that morning. Each of them still exhausted. I made a great show of cooking and offering blueberry or apple pancakes. I was trying to induce a laugh and I played on the sisterly competitive sport their Aunt Darlene and I enjoyed. I boasted that I was 'besting' their pancake menu cooked by Aunt Darlene the day before.

I served my juicy, but irregular shaped hotcakes. They were not perfect circles like Aunt

Darlene's, the accountant. I'm sure hers had the perfect circumference of the mathematical pi! I laughed, and joked. Mine did taste good.

I remember teasing Jeff. He had chosen to cut the grass today. He was riding around on the lawn mower. I said I would clean the house to prepare for the company that would arrive. He agreed this was a good idea. I teased that Kathy's parents would indeed be pleased to see a freshly cut front yard. They wouldn't mind sleeping on the clean half side of the master bed!

I tried to remove sad memories for Jeff; like her shampoo and pink razors still in the bathroom, little things. The guys brought up the daybed and reset it in the computer room. I rested my bags recklessly around the room. I put her cards and mementos in a closet. Making the room different was easier on the family.

Now neighbourhood men, Len and Jeff were on the porch chairs outside. Mom came over and joined me in cleaning. It was good to be busy. Feeling a little mischievous, I locked the men out of the house while Mom and I cleaned. Feeling guilty, I eventually opened the door to check on them and said, "If you need to use the washroom, there are some good trees down by the lakeshore." The men only laughed. They were enjoying companionship and the support they gave to each other. Later, Jeff laughingly told me that he had a house key in his pocket the whole time! I 'slapped him upside the head for this!' Laughing.

Darlene had driven home to pick up her girls and husband Wolf. They would be back tomorrow, Friday.

It was decided that 'Visitation' would be Friday. The funeral would be Saturday. A luncheon after. The 'Engagement Social' for my nephew would go on Saturday night, as planned.

Mom was stronger today. I was proud of her.

Food and condolences came from the neighbours today—lots of it.

Finished with our cleaning, Mom went home. I said that Jamie would be arriving soon, and that both of us would move into the Dungeon. I waited with Jeff and David outside on the sunny porch. Around 8:00 p.m., Brian came out. He said that Erin and Wyman were asleep, exhausted still. I offered the guys a drink.

Jamie arrived! Blissful hugs!

We all had another drink, Black Russians; Kahula, vodka and milk. Mine tasted good. We kibitzed, talked and shared. I must have filled up my drink again. It was time to grab my suitcases and move over to Mom's. As we left, I felt 'tipsy.'

We settled into Mom's house but I needed some time with my husband! We drove down to the doggy beach and parked. It reminded me of Donna and Jeff's dating days when the nostalgic 'parking/necking' term was 'going to watch the Submarine Races.' I had told Mom and Len not to wait up as we were going to watch the 'Submarine Races.' They laughed and understood.

My poor husband then allowed me to cry, shake, vent, be hysterical in my tears and also dealt with my being 'tipsy' from the drinks we had earlier! Boy, they hit me! Hours later and many hugs later, my husband settled me back at Mom's and put his rag doll wife to bed. It was now in the wee hours.

14

September 19th, Friday

We made it through Visitation in the afternoon on Friday and again in the evening. Victoria Place neighbours again providing supper. I was proud of Erin helping to prepare this feast. Relatives joined us: Auntie Joan, Uncle John, Faith, Bruce, Darlene and Wolf, and their two beautiful girls, Jenny and Amanda, Mom, and Len. The Reiners brought sleeping bags and would stay at Mom's. Auntie Marion would stay on the upstairs living-room couch for the night. She would help support Mom again, in grief again; Sisters. Uncle Gord and Scott, their son, had booked a hotel.

We were home from the visitation by 10:00 p.m. Donna had looked prettier when Faith and

I prepared her. Her hair had been wrong, curled under instead of flipped up…

I remained having to write my Eulogy. The service was at 11:00 a.m. the next morning. I talked over some ideas with Darlene and Wolf. Jeff had said I needed to include our Prayer for Donna, written by Auntie Marion's and her friend. Jamie and I left for the Submarine Races and doggy beach again. Jamie helped me organize my thoughts.

My niece Jenny had said, "It's like cramming for a school essay, then your thoughts fall into place and you get in the 'Zone.'" I had found my Zone…We got home at 3:00 a.m. I put Jamie to bed while I typed my Eulogy. Darlene had told me that if my Eulogy was typed and I was too tearful to read it, the minister would read it on my behalf. I typed until 5:00 a.m. while the household slept.

15

September 20th, Saturday

I woke later that morning. Amanda and Wolf helped me print my "document." I told them not to read it.

I asked Darlene to come to The Dungeon and listen to me read my Eulogy. I was quickly reading, as we couldn't be late for the service! With tears in her eyes, Darlene said it was beautiful! She had given me the courage and confidence to indeed read this Eulogy for Donna. I went upstairs. Mom was sitting in 'her' chair by the window. Ready to go. I quietly whispered to her that Darlene was crying, so please, look after her too!

My husband had coached me. Don't rush; just say what you need to say. After all, it's not like people would leave! His coaching had also given me confidence.

The service was beautiful. I sat with the family, beside David. Bless his heart. He told me that he wanted me beside him in the family pew. I also needed to be there.

My Uncle Gord spoke, as only a loving uncle could. At past family occasions, Uncle Gord was always relegated this task, speaking at Donna and Jeff's wedding, and other weddings. We had teamed up at happier occasions as "speakers" and bonded again, performing this duty.

He spoke of Donna being his flower girl at his own wedding. Donna and Jeff had chosen that same date for their own wedding, October 19th. This year, they would have been married for thirty-five years. My uncle also told us about a poem Donna had emailed to them years before called 'The Dash.' It explained that your life is from a birth date to a death date, and there is a 'Dash' between. The poem continued to say, 'It doesn't matter what you own or how you spend your cash, your life is measured by the quality of love and living which is represented by the 'Dash.'

The church was full. Victoria Place had come to show their respect, as well as every aunt, uncle, brother, sister, cousin and their children. All were there. Wow! I took an Ativan and walked up to the pulpit. It was now my turn to speak.

I started slowly, but my voice became stronger, as I went on…I needed to say my words.

> Hello. I'm Denise Rodda, Donna's baby sister. Donna always made me feel special, loved, and she was ALWAYS there if I needed her, through childhood and adult life.

The congregation listened…

> I hope I do the honour of being asked to eulogise her life the justice I feel this is due. How can you summarize a lifetime??? Everyone here has been touched by Donna in their own unique way. She fought cancer with grace and determination: Surpassed all medical "odds" by years. She loved being a sister, mother, wife and especially a granny. She deserves a good eulogy; I love her 'So Much.' Growing up they called us the "Three D's": Donna, Darlene, Denise. The three sisters! Our own aunts or grandparents would often get the D name mixed up. Our grandfather just called us all Shirley…don't ask me why Shirley!
>
> Should any of us had been a boy, we would have been named the D word—David—we were told.

Having been six years my senior, my sister Donna thought of me as her baby doll.

She was the little mother from an early age.

We are fortunate to have had a wonderful family oriented childhood. Family Christmases and holidays with cousins and aunts and uncles. Grandmother Ashworth's traditional holiday dinners with lots of family crowded into her small Toronto home.

Summertime fun included Travel Traile-ring. Again often with cousins, aunts and uncles and grandmothers. Donna and I rode with Mom and trailered our boat, while Darlene rode with Dad and the travel trailer.

Always looking after her younger sisters, being the "Mother," Donna usually had the responsibility of leading Darlene and I to the Community Washrooms, before bedtime. One time at a particularly "FROG" infested trailer park I was upset and crying, Sure I STEPPED ON, AND SQUISHED a FROG while on this journey! Donna INSISTED I did NOT, in order to comfort me and quiet me. I know to this day, even though I was likely four years old, I know I DID STEP ON AND SQUISH THAT FROG!!!

At the cottages, again with family of all assortments joining in, we enjoyed swimming, bonfires, and fishing. Singing "Joy to the World and Joy to the Fishes in the DEEP BLUE SEA!" was the first fishing strategy we learned!!! Mom's special fish fries were a treat.

Water fights with cousins included buckets of water thrown at each other from the dock, yard, and even out to Cousin Greg in his "Little Green Boat." We didn't have fancy water guns in those days, but we did have fun.

The "Three D's" grew to be the perfect water-ski team. Darlene and I, the avid skiers; Donna was our reliable boat driver, so we had the legal requirements of skier, driver, and spotter. It was great!

She met Jeff while working as a dental assistant. He saw her in the parking lot, and then walked into his dental appointment only to see her there too! In his words, she was so beautiful he wasn't going to leave until he had a date!!!

That was the start of the McCauley Family as Jeff and Donna saw each other non-stop since that first Ontario Place date.

Jeff joined the family then too. Being eleven years old at the time, I remember he and Donna, driving me and girlfriends to Brownie meetings and making sea weed monsters out of Darlene and I, Yes mostly Jeff. I remember sneaking peaks at them kissing goodnight at the doorway!!!

Our late Father enjoyed keeping Jeff on his toes by giving him many household painting and odd projects to do. Wanting to get on Dad's best side, Jeff humbly and with a smile, did all Dad asked of him, if the promise of Donna's love might be the rewards for this. By age 13, I made it known if Donna changed her mind about Jeff for any reason, I would marry Jeff!!!

They married young, Donna eighteen, Jeff twenty-two, then moved to London Ontario to be nearer to the family. Sunday dinners at Mom's were a must for family orientated Donna.

Wolfgang, my next brother-in law joined the family and more fun was had. When she had her first born child, a boy, Donna and Jeff named him David. She gave my mother the gift of "Finally" having her David in the family. The Boy D name she had picked out. She gave me the gift of being Godparent to David when I was only seventeen years old.

Donna stayed at home to mother and focus on her child and husband. Sensing David's desire for a sibling when he invented imaginary play friends; Racoons, Donna and Jeff had their second child, Erin.

Erin was the apple of her mother's eye. Her own Baby Doll. I remember her long blonde hair bouncing, she was always dressed so sweetly too.

Jeff was transferred to Kentucky when the kids were just starting their teen age years.

Ya'll know, the four Canadians made the adjustment well: Donna decorating an outstandingly beautiful house. She became quite an expert golfer with now longstanding friends. She became an email "junkie" in order to keep in touch with family and friends. She catered solely to her family: driving children to swim meets, welcoming their friends into her home—Mothering.

Eventually she returned to work as an Orthodontic Assistant. Again showing her abundant motherly love for children—making the difficult job of applying braces to children a fun one!

Doing their laundry and making care packages of peanut butter cookies when both her children were at University eventually evolved.

Jeff was then transferred to Texas: now a core family of two. She surprised me with her adventurous spirit, but of course, she would follow Jeff anywhere!! They enjoyed exploring the area together with frequent weekend outings.

Her tragic terminal illness began here so Jeff returned his Donna to Canada, to be near family, and her mother at Victoria Place. A wonderful community where a loving nature must be a requirement for the purchase of housing.

In the past two weeks of her illness, we must thank many neighbours for their God-Send gifts of meals and their emotional support.

Our Mother, Ruth, was devoted, as was her husband, Jeff, to supporting Donna with her fight of this terrible disease.

Donna's battle and death by cancer has saved me and my sister Darlene's lives.

She was found to be genetically positive for this illness. No fault can be laid on her.

Because of this the world of Ontario Health has "Opened Up" to our family. I was diagnosed also genetically positive and have participated in two medical research studies for ovarian and breast cancer. And we have taken preventive medical measures offered to us so we should never need endure the same terrible fate Donna has.

I feel we should all learn from this. To advise our doctor of any family medical "notorious" history while at an early age so prevention can be attained!

I also feel she has saved every future ancestor: daughters, nieces, cousins, and their children: male and female will never be afflicted or die so young from this genetic predisposition. Now—because of her.

Donna fought cancer for twelve years. She beat the odds as she was determined to live to see her children settled.

She was thrilled her son was recently engaged to a beautiful Kentucky woman. Here with her family today for their first visit to share this joy and sorrow with the McCauley family and friends.

She surpassed expectations and lived to see her 'Pride and Joy,' Erin's first born child, Wyman. To now be a "GRANNY" as she had dreamed of this. We have taken Brian into the family heart now too.

In the past weeks she solidified the relationships in our family again while we provided care for her. Together drawing on each others strengths. She passed into Heaven gently at home with her house full of family and loved ones. This forged bonds which can never be broken. She can now watch down on all her family, no earthly distances will interfere. Donna is truly a 'part' of all of us here. Our tears are for sadness we feel at not having her physically with us. Loneliness for her.

We owe Donna, who proved such a strong determined fighter for life, to continue to enjoy people, especially family and children, to enjoy laughter... to enjoy flowers and gardens and nature, animals and pets, especially cats. As she fought to enjoy these! Enjoy Life!

She will be here with us all now.

On her death bed at home, she told me she loved me SOOO MUCH and I told her I loved her SOO MUCH.

We were BIG SIS AND LITTLE SIS and we still are.

Please join me in a prayer my aunt brought to us, which we leaned on for support during these last weeks with Donna.

Heavenly Father,

You look after us and continually hold us in Your arms. Your strength can carry us through any situation. We lean on You now Lord as we come together and Lift Donna up before You. May Your Grace light her Life. May Your Peace, the peace of God that passes all understanding, saturate Donna's body, mind and Spirit. Please surround Donna with Your ever-present Angels to comfort and strengthen her. We pray for healing and freedom from pain. And Father, please be with us all and guide us on the journey. In Jesus' name we pray. Amen. Thank you.

I walked exhausted back to my seat…

My husband Jamie was a pallbearer, along with Cousin Wayne, Cousin Scott, Wolfgang and Reg, Joe, and Jerry McCauley, Jeff's brothers. Kathy's father is a minister in Kentucky. He was gracious enough to speak also. He was quite tickled I had teasingly added the 'Ya'll' within my speech and he played on this also.

The service was now over.

Now the visiting and reuniting with family began at the luncheon. I made a point of asking relatives to come back this evening to the Victoria Place clubhouse to join us for David and Kathy's engagement social. To please help us fulfill Donna's last wish. We needed to continue to support each other through this occasion!

We had a few hours before David and Kathy's social. I spoke with Darlene, and she took care of me yet again saying, "just go away." The

Reiner family, with the help of the McCauley family would decorate and organize this function. I took her advice and Jamie and I found the 'Submarine Races' again at a secluded waterside boat launch. I napped in the sun. Before going back to Mom's house to dress, we went to the doggy beach again. I had intended to go for a swim to revitalize.

Someone was there! Donna's best friend. We said our hellos and Ann pointed out the clouds she'd been watching. "Don't they resemble angels?" Yes, they did. Ann told me that she and Donna would sit at this picnic table to rest on their walks. Donna would hum and sing. I don't know what songs she sang, but it was nice to hear her singing. Ann then shared her special *Blessing* with me. At the funeral, a funeral card with Donna's picture, her smiling, had fallen and was looking at Ann. Ann felt that Donna was beside her during the whole service. Leave it to my sister! With her curious mind, her spirit would want to see her own service. A perfect place to watch, beside her friend! I feel my sister would have been pleased.

Back at Mom's house, Len and Mom were the only ones left at the household. Mom was weepy. Jamie and I dressed for David and Kathy's social. I wore green and gray and my pink breast cancer heart pendant. My Mom told me that green represents ovarian cancer. We encouraged Mom and Len to come with us. "It's not a party, its Donna's last wish! It's a further chance to gain support with the family. We need to make Donna proud by uniting with Kathy's family." Tearfully they joined us.

At the Victoria Place Clubhouse doorway, Mom was consumed with hugs from relatives. Donna had perhaps known that this support would be positive.

The buffet table was laden with the flower arrangements from the service. Donna's presence there too! There was no music, nor alcohol. Respectfully, Kathy's father said a few words, a *Blessing*. Wolf said a toast to the new couple. The room was then alive with conversation and hugs. Later, it was said that this was truly a family reunion. Surely, under any other circumstances, not as many people would have been able to attend. Donna loved this, I'm sure!

16

September 21st, Sunday

I was exhausted and needed to recuperate. Jamie knew I would not rest here at Mom's house, as I would drive myself to help others. We departed for home the next morning. As we had two vehicles to drive back to Sault Ste. Marie, Jamie was worried about me driving for ten hours. He knew I was exhausted. He insisted that I drive behind him as we drove from Tim Horton's Coffee Shop to Tim Horton's Coffee Shop, back home. I had Donna's stuffed doggy toy on my lap. It gave me peace and strength.

I was desperately tired and purchased a 'trucker five hour alertness drink.' Yuk! It tasted terrible but I was now packed with energy.

As we were driving into the sunset towards Sault Ste. Marie, a pink glow was on the horizon with only a very few clouds in site. Then I saw it! To my skyward left, there appeared a small rainbow. My angel, Donna, must have been watching over me, my safety. I watched as I drove and pointed out my car window in hopes that Jamie would also see it. This *Blessing!* Then the small rainbow disappeared. I reached for my camera and sat it on the dash. I snapped some pictures and hoped perhaps the rainbow would appear again.

I looked at the pictures later that week. Amongst them was the picture of the highway, and the surrounding traffic headlights. The headlights had blurred in the image. Amazingly, the blurred images looked like Angels with trails coming down from the Heavens. I had asked Donna to be my special Angel, and she is! I am *Blessed!*

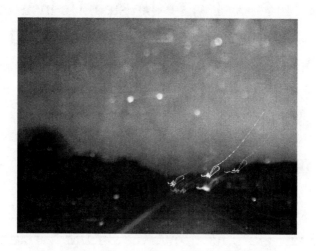

Epilogue

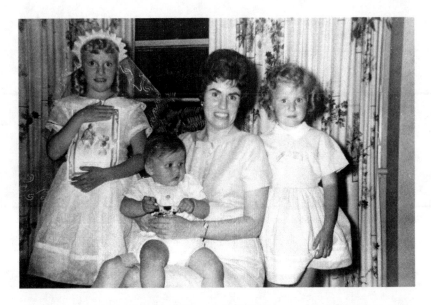

Aunt Joan with the "Three D's," Donna, Darlene, and Denise. Our Genetic Tree—each has been affected by familial cancer.

The Plea!

Ten months later, we still grieve. My Angel has also provided me with many more *Blessings* in life.

The next family get together was in November, in Kentucky, David and Kathy's wedding. I could not stop the flow of tears. The Star Gazer Lily, at the alter, was in memory of Donna. It was surrounded by white trailing roses to represent others revered and deceased family members...grandparents. This was a testament to Donna's *Blessing* on this wedding.

Throughout the following months, I have accumulated a collection of angels. All of them given to me for assorted reasons. I am trying to become accustomed with having my 'Big Sis Angel' with me all of the time.

We grieve, then heal, then grieve again. Through this, we must always recognise and count our *Blessings*.

Donna's battle and death by cancer has saved me and my sister Darlene's lives. She was found to be genetically positive, BRAC2 positive, for this illness. No fault can be laid on her.

Donna's first episode with breast cancer was in Kentucky. She opted for a lumpectomy as the cancer had been caught at a good time. Breast cancer is where breast tissue and nodes become diseased, defective, start destroying cells and try to thrive and metastasize, spread throughout the body. Those who are genetically positive, for breast cancer, also have a 30% chance of getting ovarian cancer and usually at a young adult age. Some other increased predispositions exist for genetic carriers of both sexes. Ovarian cancer is deadly and harder to stop from spreading. The estrogens from the breast play a factor.

Now comes the 'What ifs?'

"What if" someone had realized upon Donna's first cancer diagnosis and treatment, that our family history held an overwhelming number of young deaths or occurrences with breast cancer? Would Donna have been genetically tested then? Would her treatment have been more medically aggressive? Would she have been offered preventive health interventions as I have been? Interventions I have taken.

Can we not all learn to pass on the most precious gift of 'Health' to our loved ones? I plead with all those who read this, Donna's Legacy of Blessings, to please write down everything you can remember regarding your sisters, brothers, mothers, fathers, aunt, uncles, grandparents, cousins, and great-grandparents: health concerns, diabetes; heart or kidney problems; cancers; allergies; asthma, etc. Make a genealogy of health concerns. Family history repeats itself! Swap your version of this health genealogy with other family members. I implore you to do this for your children and their children's children! This awareness will save our lives and ensure our quality of life is at its maximum. If we know: If we know at an *early age*!

We can take medical action to prevent, treat and heal disease. Genetic studies of familial genes are just one example. BRAC 2 is a known cancer causing defects in our chromosomes, passed down at birth. There is a 50/50 chance that this will occur if one parent is positive for this gene.

Other genes are medically recognised in relationship to colon cancer, alzheimer's, and Down syndrome. Medical research is trying to learn more. So we can learn. Society can no longer afford our health care systems. What a savings, if we were all healthier? Learning from the personal health genealogies we can create!

If only everyone had their own "Family Legacy for Donna": their Health Genealogy. After being diagnosed with deadly ovarian cancer, my sister Donna underwent extensive treatment. She remised many times. She adapted her life the best way she could, trying to love and enjoy when she was able.

What would it have been like if we had access to this health genealogy when we were still in our formative years? When we begin making and forming lifestyles? In our twenties?

If Donna had known then, could she have prolonged her life? Society's young adults can now prolong their lives, by listening to this plea to be aware of your health history. Society's young adults could learn to support each other in their life choices, for health prevention. Would Donna have taken the advised prophylactic/preventive treatments I have undergone? If she had known before she was stricken with breast cancer? While in her 20's or even her 30's? Could she have accessed preventive treatments as I have? If only she had known! My cancer risk factors are 3% now. I have enjoyed medical Preventive Intervention!

If we knew heart disease was rampant in our family history, would we avoid smoking and take up a "cardio" exercise? Perhaps tailor our careers to ensure daily exercise and longevity?! Become a mailman?! Would we have our yearly physical examinations and inform our doctors of our health genealogies, every time we seek medical attention! Would we do something as simple, as avoiding salt in our diets, prolonging the onset of high blood pressure/hypertension many years! Or avoid sugar in our diets from birth, if we should have a strong diabetic history? Thus potentially delaying this disease's onset! What diseases and conditions did our relatives live with? And die with?! Would we attend genetic counselling appointments yearly, to learn the latest in health research? Diagnostics and preventions and studies! So many, many opportunities, IF we only knew!

Please *Bless* your family by making a health genealogy; *Legacy for Donna*. If only she had known.

THE END

Donna, her family, and those involved in this tragic story, are pleased to share this personal natural part of our lives, "If it shall help 'only one person.' We pray that one Person is You!"